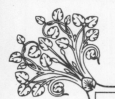

The Book of Home Remedies and Herbal Cures

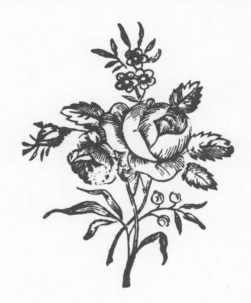

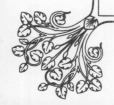

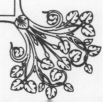

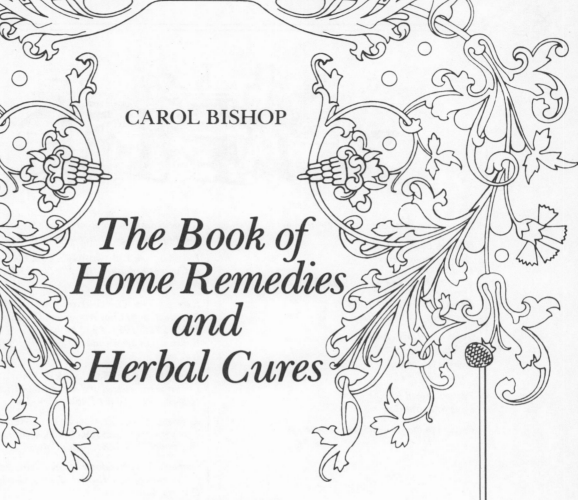

CAROL BISHOP

The Book of
Home Remedies
and
Herbal Cures

A Jonathan-James Book

OCTOPUS
MAYFLOWER

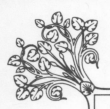
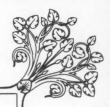

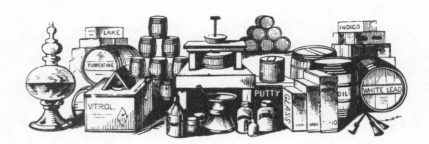

This edition first published in 1979 by

Octopus Books Limited
59 Grosvenor Street
London W1
© 1979 Jonathan-James Books

Paperback   0 7064 1088 2
Hardback   0 7064 1069 6

Jonathan-James Books
5 Sultan Street
Toronto Ontario
Canada M5S 1L6

Editor: Ingrid Philipp Cook
Design: Brant Cowie

Printed in the United States of America

Grateful acknowledgment is made for permission to use the following copyrighted material.

Excerpts from Bill Wannan's Folk Medicine, *Hill of Content Publishing Co. Pty Ltd. Melbourne, Australia.*

Excerpts from The Foxfire Book, *edited with an Introduction by Eliot Wigginton. Copyright © 1968, 1969, 1970, 1971, 1972 by the Foxfire Fund, Inc. Reprinted by permission of Doubleday & Company, Inc.*

Illustrations from Handbook of Plant and Floral Ornament, *selected and arranged by Richard G. Hatton, 1960, Dover Publications, Inc.*

Apothecaries Weights from Instant Metric Conversion, *Bryan Ross & K.V. Dyck Ltd, Vancouver V6B 3Z8, British Columbia, Canada*

Glossary of Herbs adapted from Herb Seed Catalogue, *© Otto Richter & Sons, Goodwood, Ontario, Canada L0C 1A0*

Excerpts from Texas Folk Medicine *by John Q. Anderson, Encino Press, Austin, Texas. By permission, Texas Folklore Society.*

Excerpts from An Historical Almanac of Canada *by Lena Newman reprinted by permission of The Canadian Publishers, McClelland and Stewart Limited, Toronto.*

Every reasonable effort has been made to ascertain copyright. If we have unwittingly infringed copyright in any excerpt or illustration reproduced in this book we tender our sincerest apologies and will be glad of the opportunity, upon being satisfied as to the owner's title, to pay an appropriate fee as if we had been able to obtain prior permission.

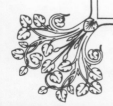
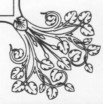

To Michael

Acknowledgments

This book would not have been possible without the love, patience and encouragement of Michael McIvor. My appreciation to editor Ingrid Philipp Cook for her friendship and guidance. A special thanks to the Australian media which publicized my request for remedies and to all the wonderful people who took the time to write to me. My thanks also to the many librarians I consulted, Marjory Morphy at the Academy of Medical Archives in Toronto, provincial and state archivists, and especially Marion Schoon, reference librarian at Harvard's Widener Library.
CAROL BISHOP

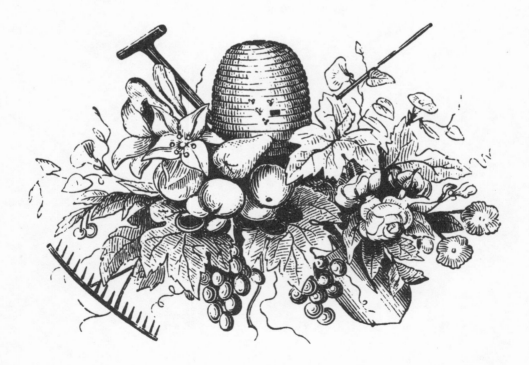

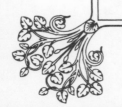
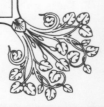

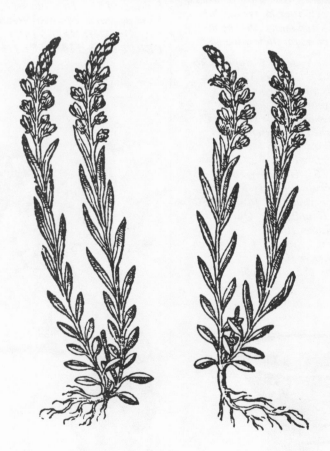

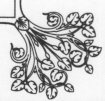

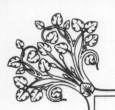

Contents

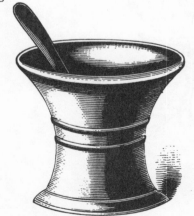

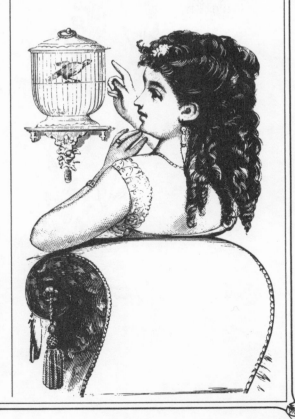

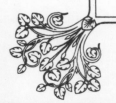

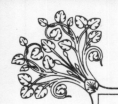

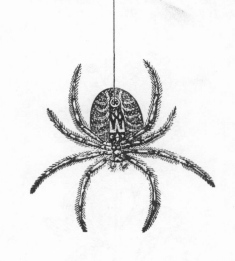

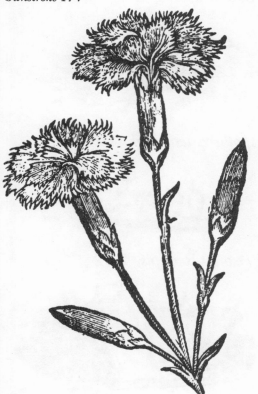

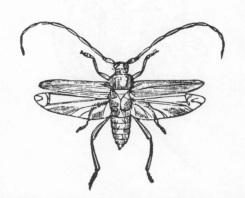

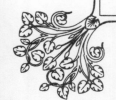

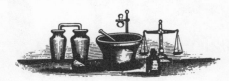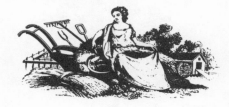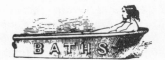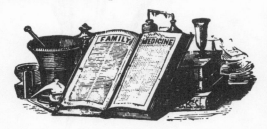
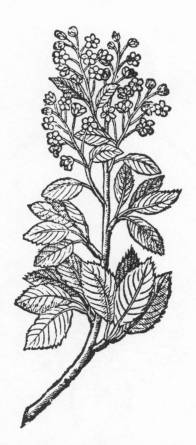

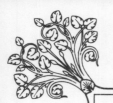

The Book of Home Remedies and Herbal Cures

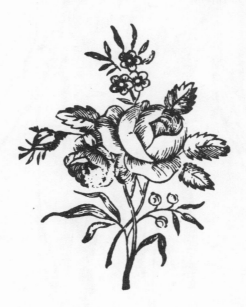

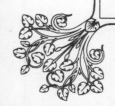
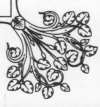

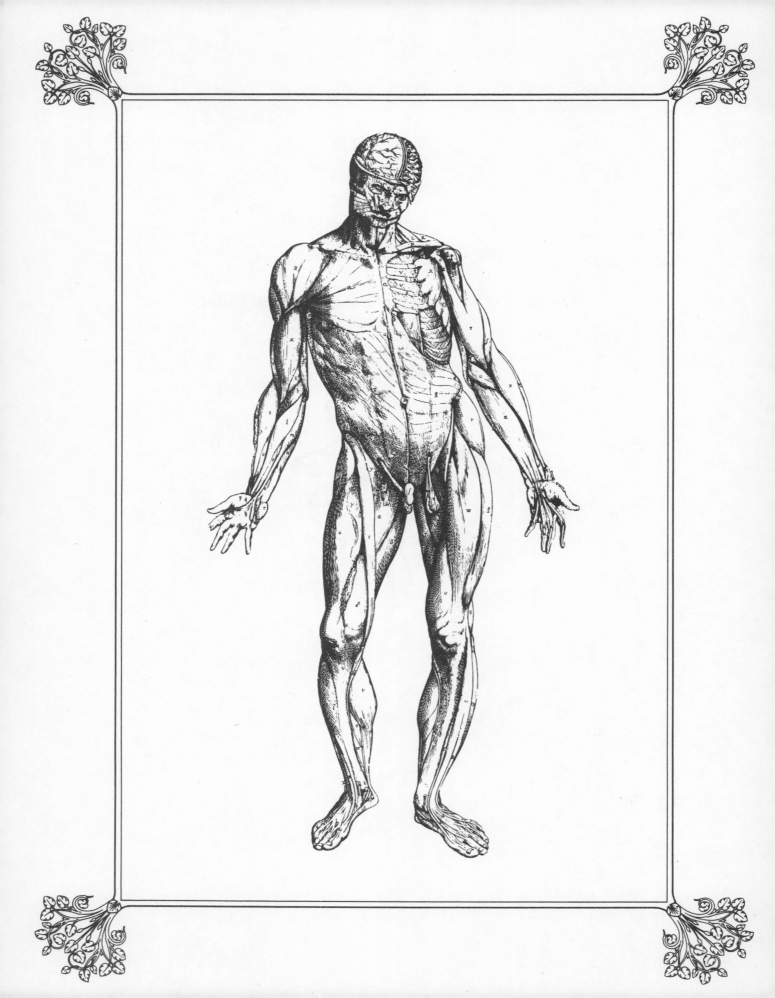

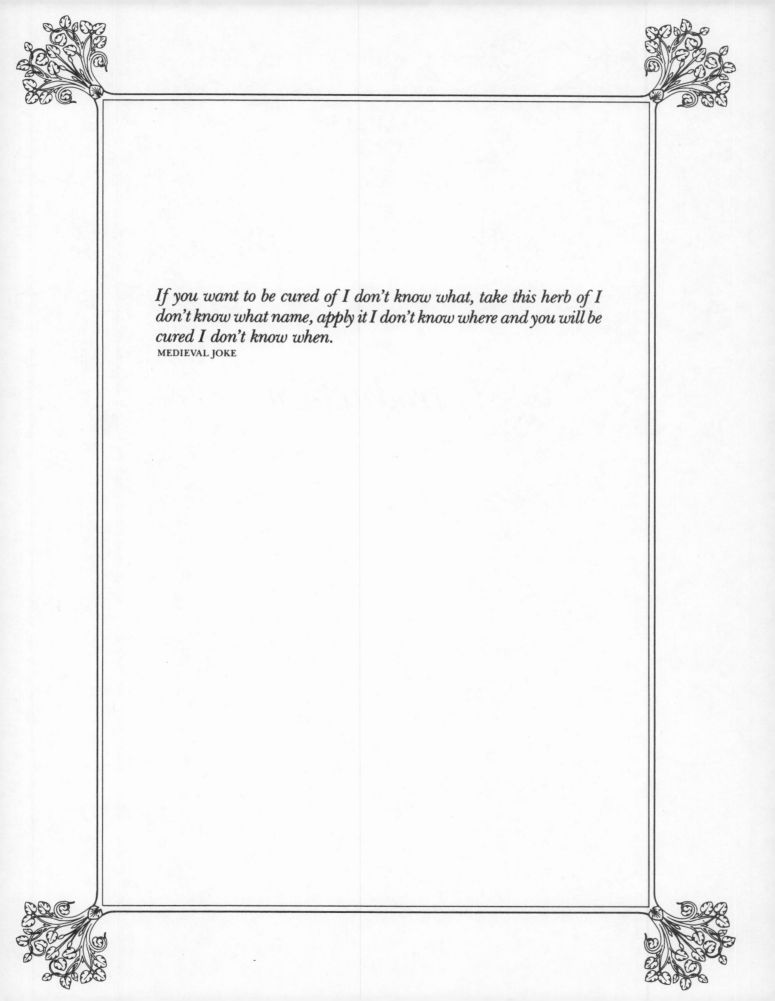

If you want to be cured of I don't know what, take this herb of I don't know what name, apply it I don't know where and you will be cured I don't know when.
MEDIEVAL JOKE

CHAPTER
ONE

Introduction

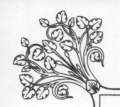

Home remedies are a curiosity to most of us; a quaint collection of old wives' superstitions used by uneducated and simple rural folk. We tend to forget that these so-called granny recipes saved many of our ancestors in times when doctors were few and far between and viewed with distrust. As our society has become more advanced, we have traded our proud self-sufficiency for a multitude of specialists, each trained to cater to a specific need. Modern technology has certainly eased our existence, but it has also put us at the mercy of the knowledge of others. This sense of helplessness and dependency has driven some to attempt to return to a less complex and more self-reliant world. As the commonsense practices of those who lived in that kind of world are rediscovered, we find increased admiration for our forebears — especially for the women who took the role of mother, wife, doctor, nursemaid, midwife, herbalist, druggist, beautician, laundress and cleaner, to name but a few.

While THE BOOK OF HOME REMEDIES AND HERBAL CURES *has been put into chapters and the complaints arranged in alphabetical order for easy reference, this system would not be found in the old housewifery or cookery books. In those books there was no systematic order. For example, in one 17th century household book, I found recipes for almond custard, a tickling cough or rhume and ragou of veal, all on the same page. Whenever the lady of the house came across a useful recipe, she would copy it down in her diary and these books would pass from mother to daughter, each in turn copying their recipes into the family book. I am awed by how or when these busy women ever found the time to prepare complicated beauty potions and hygiene products, such as those found in the Beauty chapter, for their own use.*

Whenever I came across one of these family books in an archive and turned the pages, I wondered about its owners. Often there were pages devoted to the practice of the alphabet. With paper being at such a premium, these books would double as copybooks for young girls learning to write. In the later diaries, newspaper clippings with household tips and recipes would be tucked into the pages. These books held all the acquired wisdom collected over a lifetime of caring for a family.

This tradition of doctor books began when the English ladies of the manor took over the responsibility of tending the ill, a function previously fulfilled by the monasteries. The duties of a lady included growing all the herbs and plants or 'simples' required for various cures and her care extended to all her husband's tenants. Of course, the peasants also had their own medical wisdom passed down through the ages by word of mouth.

It is this oral tradition that we are most in danger of losing with our modern communication systems. It is startling to realize we may have

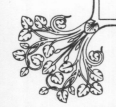
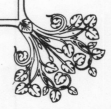

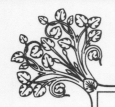

with us today the last generation to possess the knowledge transmitted by such an oral tradition. People of that generation can still tell us stories of having their wounds bound with cobwebs, or wearing a piece of camphor around their necks all winter to ward off colds, or swallowing diabolical potions which may or may not have cured their stomach aches. My request for home remedies from newspaper readers in Australia brought a flood of testimony from many older people with vivid memories of how they managed to survive childhood without professional medical attention. Many native peoples, who were forced to give up their traditional medicine men, fear that the wisdom accumulated over hundreds of years has been lost forever.

This is not to suggest in any way that we should spurn or ridicule the tremendous advances made by modern medicine. However, we have tended to deride home remedies as old granny superstitions when in fact, many of them had great practical value. Neither am I suggesting we reject modern science and technology. But rather, I am chiding all of us to perhaps stop and see if we really need that advertised 'wonder' product when plain old soap and water or baking soda may work just as well. Maybe you will even be inspired to cultivate a few traditional medicinal herbs by the informative chapter on making an indoor herbal garden, written by Ingrid Cook. It would certainly be carrying on the tradition of the English ladies of the manor.

I have tried to be faithful to the spellings used in the original sources for the remedies and have attempted to explain the unfamiliar terms and ingredients. Some have defeated inquiry. Measurements in some cases are less than specific; my favourite being the pugil, which is a little handful or a big pinch. And I am at a loss to suggest where you can find such ingredients as rind from paradise or a swallow's womb.

Obviously these remedies are not recommended to replace professional medical knowledge. THE BOOK OF HOME REMEDIES AND HERBAL CURES is meant to be enjoyed as an entertaining catalogue showing us how our ancestors coped with their aches, pains, vanities and household problems. I also hope this collection of remedies has, in its own small way, helped to preserve and pass on a legacy of knowledge we are in danger of losing forever.

Carol Bishop
March, 1979

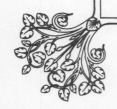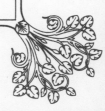

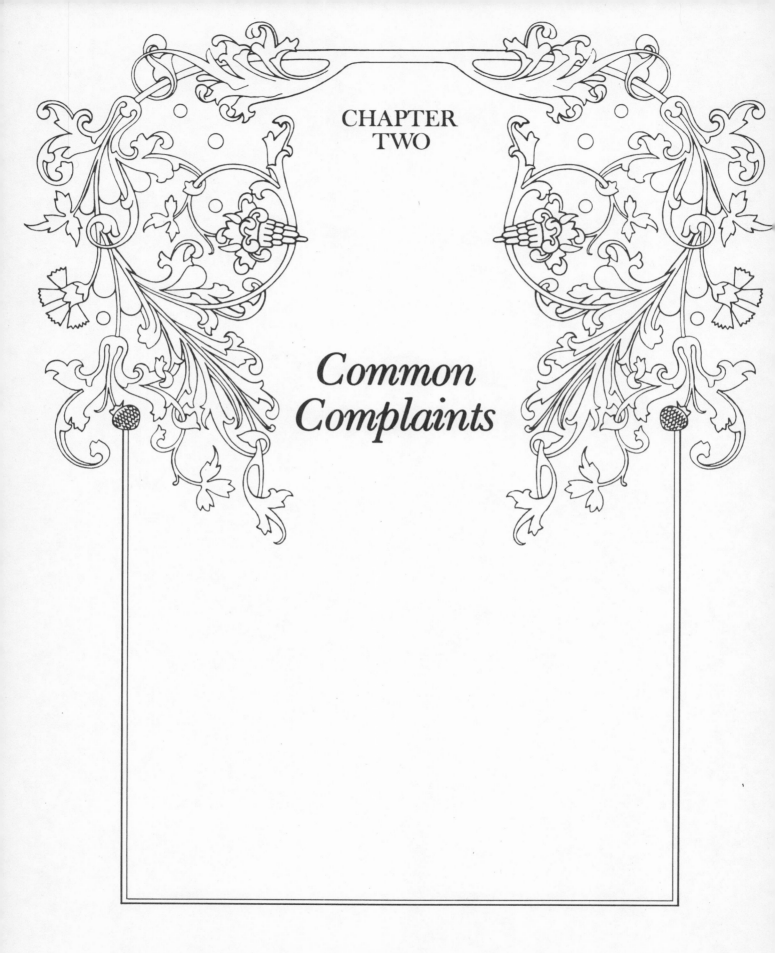

CHAPTER TWO

Common Complaints

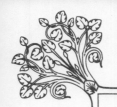
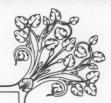

Although our lives bear little resemblance to the existence of our forefathers, some human conditions have proved constant. Over the ages, we have managed to eradicate some diseases, control others and we now successfully treat maladies which would have killed us in the past. However, we can still commiserate with our ancestors over headaches, colds and coughs, rheumatism, hiccups and most certainly over the agonies of heartbreak. Naturally, we have always tried to find ways of relieving our pain and suffering, and although today's doctors look askance at most of the so-called "quackery" from the past, many home remedies had a sound medical basis and have stood the test of time.

We tend to forget that it has only been in the last one hundred years that synthetic drugs have been produced and at the beginning of the 20th century, natural remedies using plants and herbs had a leading place in the official pharmacopias of the world. Many modern medicines actually contain plant or herbal ingredients which have been used for countless generations. We get penicillin and many of the antibiotics from moulds and lichens (the Egyptians used mouldy bread as a healing agent); digitalis, a blood pressure lowering agent, from foxglove; atropine with its anaesthetic properties from belladona and the list goes on and on. Often our ancestors used a plant without scientific knowledge of why it worked. They just knew that it cured the patient.

These cherished home remedies passed from generation to generation by word of mouth or were copied into ledgers which went by such names as still-room books, doctor books or common place books. When printing made commercial books and newspapers widely accessible, volumes of recipes and herbals became best sellers. One of the more popular of the British herbalists was Nicholas Culpeper (1616–54) whose best known book, The English Physician, had five reprintings before 1698. Culpeper incited the wrath of the College of Physicians by translating and publishing books of medical knowledge for the common man, thus intruding in the doctors' privileged and lucrative domain. Culpeper's reciprocal contempt for the College of Physicians is apparent in his writings. 'Bees are industrious and go abroad to gather honey from each plant and flower, but drones lie at home and eat up what the bees have taken pains for; just so do the college of physicians lie at home and domineer and suck out the sweetness of other men's honour and studies, themselves as ignorant in the knowledge of herbs as a child of four years old,' he said.

Almost a century later, another Englishman, Reverend John Wesley (1703–91), founder of the Methodist Church, published a book of home remedies to give advice and relief to his followers. It was called The Primitive Physick – An Easy and Natural Way of Curing Most

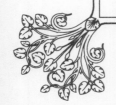
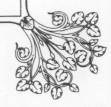

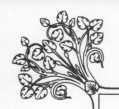

Diseases. *Cold baths seemed to have been his favourite 'cure-all' for everything from convulsions to tetanus. Reverend Wesley was likely a better preacher than amateur doctor as many of his suggested cures were quite useless. In addition, he dismissed the one effective cure for malaria at the time, Peruvian bark, as 'extremely dangerous'. However his little book of remedies was very popular, enjoyed many reprintings and was often quoted by newspapers and other books.*

One of the reverend's admirers was Dr Alvin Chase, an American who published a series of medical home remedy books beginning in the 1860s. Dr Chase, who informed his readers that he began in the retail drug and grocery business, published small pamphlets of remedies which were expanded into several books. He later branched into the profitable field of patent medicines. Maybe some of you still remember Dr Chase's Dyspeptic Cordial—$1.00 a bottle—and Dr Chase's Liver and Anti-Bilious Pills—25¢ a box?

Just as the remedies passed from generation to generation and were carried to new countries, so too were many of the plants transported. A number of weeds and herbs we take for granted as being indigenous were actually brought by conquerors to plant in their physic gardens. The Romans introduced Mediterranean plants to northern Europe and Britain. Similarly, in the 10th and 11th centuries, the monks brought exotics from the great abbeys of France and Italy to England for their herbal gardens and later the Puritans brought seeds and slips to the New World to provide a ready supply of ingredients for their Old World cures. Most expeditions to the Americas and the Far East included a botanist who was charged with finding new drugs and effective native cures. Probably one of the biggest debts Europe owes the New World came in the 17th century when the Spanish Jesuits learned of the fever-reducing properties of the cinchona or Peruvian bark from the South American natives. This natural quinine saved millions of Europeans from death by malaria.

All this is not to deny that many of the remedies and their ingredients are dangerous, sometimes lethal. Often the remedy was worse than the disease. A tragic case in point was the widespread use of calomel, a mercury compound, administered in massive doses, especially during the American Civil war, which slowly destroyed the nervous system of the patient. Other examples are stramonium, which can paralyze the heart, sassafras, which contains a carcinogenic ingredient, or mistletoe, which contains toxic proteins which can cause both anemia and hemorrhaging in the liver and intestines. But, as I mentioned before, other remedies had a sound medical basis and happily cured the patient. Some were neither harmful nor effective, but perhaps had the same effect as the placebo pills

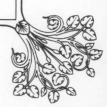

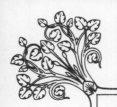

now used to convince the patient of recovery. At times a variety of remedies were tried if the disease was difficult to diagnose. And is this so different from the current practice where a doctor, baffled by a patient's symptoms, tries a series of drugs until one does the trick or the complaint has gone away of its own accord. There is a medieval joke about this approach to curing: 'If you want to be cured of I don't know what, take this herb of I don't know what name, apply it I don't know where and you will be cured I don't know when.'

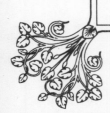
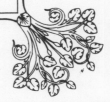

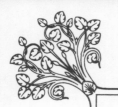

Aches and Pains

He preaches patience that never knew pain.
ENGLISH PROVERB

A RECEIPT FOR BACK-ACHE: Let a little girl under seven years, spin yarn out of flax, and make a string of it and put it around you and wear it until it comes off.
JOHN STONER'S SYMPATHY—A COLLECTION OF EXCELLENT REMEDIES AND RECIPES FOR THE CURE OF VARIOUS DISEASES OF PERSONS AND CATTLE,
OHIO, 1867

AN OINTMENT FOR ALL KINDS OF ACHES: Take gander's fat, the fat of a male cat and red boar's fat and three drams of blue wax, watercress, wormwood, the red strawberry plant and primrose. Boil them in pure spring water and when boiled stuff a gander with them and roast them at a distance from the fire. The grease issuing from it should be carefully kept in a pot. It is a valuable ointment for all kinds of aches in a man's body and it is like one that was formerly made by Hippocrates. It is proved.
OLD WELSH CURE

When John Josselyn (1638–75) arrived in New England to study the botanical species of that part of the new world, he discovered that the Indians had a similar cure using bear's fat.

FOR ACHES AND COLD SWELLINGS: The grease of a black bear is very good for aches and cold swellings. The Indians anoint themselves therewith from top to toe; which hardens them against the cold weather.
JOHN JOSSELYN, *NEW ENGLAND RARITIES,* LONDON, 1672

Black bears were at bargain prices in the 17th century, as John Josselyn explained. 'A black bear's skin heretofore was worth forty shillings, now you may have one for ten; much used by the English for beds and coverlets and by the Indians for coats.' However, because of dwindling wildlife populations, it is a very different story today. So here is a cure using 'easy-to-get' ingredients. In fact, many people would say that tobacco is too easy to get, but when it was first brought to Europe from North America, it was considered a medicine.

PAINS: Steep marigold in good cider vinegar, and frequently wash the affected parts; this will afford speedy relief; or take half a pound of tar and half a pound of tobacco, and boil them down separately to a thick substance, then simmer them together; spread a plaster, and apply it to the affected parts and it will afford immediate relief.
LADIES INDISPENSABLE ASSISTANT, NEW YORK 1851

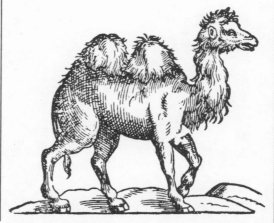

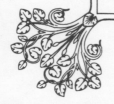

The Ladies Indispensable Assistant *had a rather long subtitle: 'Being a Companion for the Sister, Mother and Wife—A Great Variety of Valuable Recipes Forming a Complete System of Family Medicine, Thus Enabling Each Person to Become His or Her Own Physician.'*

Neuralgia, which literally means nerve pain, is used to describe pains with no discernible cause. Neuralgia could result from many problems such as overwork and anxiety, exposure to cold and damp, bruising of a nerve by a blow, or tooth decay. Some of our forebearers used these remedies to ease the pain.

KENTUCKY REMEDIES:
• Neuralgia can be cured if the sufferer will for three consecutive days take nine swallows of water after rising in the morning and before speaking.
• If you are suffering from neuralgia in the left side of the head, take a piece of red wrapping string, ignite it and sniff the smoke into the right nostril and vice versa.
FROM *KENTUCKY SUPERSTITIONS*, 1920

A FRIEND WHO suffered terrible pains from neuralgia, hearing of a noted physician in Germany who invariably cured the disease, went to him, and was permanently cured after a short sojourn. The doctor gave him the remedy, which was nothing but a poultice and tea made from our common field thistle. The leaves are macerated and used as a poultice on the parts affected, while a small quantity of the same is boiled down to the proportion of a quart to a pint and a small wineglass of the decoction drank before each meal. Our friend says he has never known it to fail in giving relief, while in almost every case it has effected a cure.
THE CANADIAN HOME COOK BOOK, 1877

This Chinese remedy may have given temporary relief, since peppermint has a very high concentration of menthol, which has a cooling effect. Because of its pleasant taste, peppermint is the most popular single herb in the world.

SUFFERERS FROM NEURALGIA may be pleased to learn from a medical correspondent of the London Lancet that: 'A few years ago, when in China, I ascertained that the natives when attacked with facial neuralgia used oil of peppermint which they lightly applied to the seat of the pain with a camel's hair pencil.'
NEWSPAPER CLIPPING FOUND IN SCRAPBOOK OF CANADIAN PIONEER

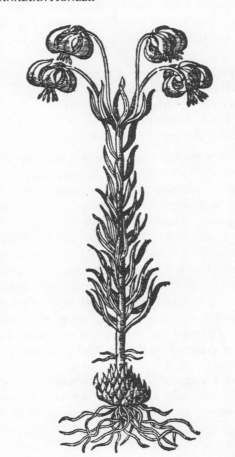

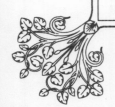
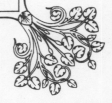

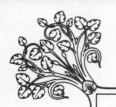

Ague

That same ague that hath made you lean.
SHAKESPEARE, *JULIUS CAESAR*

Ague traditionally has referred to any unexplainable fever, but in most cases the sufferer had malaria. The English had a charm against ague that was to be recited up the chimney by the eldest female of the family on the eve of St. Agnes. Since St. Agnes, patron saint of chastity, is honoured on January 21, the chant should be recited on the evening previous. I'm not sure if this eldest female in the family should be in the same state of grace as St. Agnes.

Tremble and go!
First day shiver and burn:
Tremble and quake!
Second day shiver the learn:
Tremble and die!
Third day never return.

I found the following cure in a book written around 1750, subtitled 'Charity made pleasant by relieving their own Family or poor neighbouring People by cheap, easy and safe remedies.' And in the introduction, there is a complaint that still rings true today: 'Physic has long been deemed an Art to be acquired but by Men of Learning only; but the Exorbitance of their Fees, and the Extravagance of Apothecaries Bills, has made Family Receipts much esteemed, more especially when they are well chosen and adopted to the Cure designed by Reason and Experience.'

FOR AN AGUE: Take a spider alive, cover it with soft crummy bread without bruising it: Let the patient swallow it fasting. This is an effectual cure, but many are set against it. It has frequently been given to people who did not know the contents and has had the desired effect.
THE HOUSEKEEPER'S POCKETBOOK—EVERYONE THEIR OWN PHYSICIAN, C. 1750

According to an Old English proverb, 'agues come on horseback, but go away on foot.' Perhaps this next recipe attempted to fight fire with fire.

TO MAKE YE HORSE DUNGE WATER: Take horse dunge and putt to it so much ale as will make it like hasty pudding and put it into your still. Then putt on ye topp one pound of treakell and a quarter pound of genger in powder, and a quarter of a pound of sweet anniseeds and so distill all these together. This water is good for women in labour and in child-bed, for agues and feavers and all distempters.
THE RECEIPT BOOK OF MRS ANN BLENCOWE, 1694

Personally, I'd rather suffer from ague than eat live spiders or drink horse-dung water. However, our ancestors had many remedies in which the ingredients were highly effective. The next two recipes will reduce fevers because they include jesuit or Peruvian bark, which contains quinine, a fever-reducing agent. It was brought back to Europe from South America by the Jesuits who learned of its medicinal properties from the natives. Peruvian bark also proves that modern medicine does not always triumph. Certain strains of malaria have built up a resistance to the modern, synthetic quinine, but continue to respond to the natural product.

AN ELECTUARY FOR INTERMITTING FEVERS: Mix one ounce of snake root with a pound of jesuits bark, both beaten into a powder and infused into as much syrup of cloves as will make it an electuary. Between the fits take about the bigness of a chestnut, and

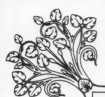

when you have repeated that about three or four days, you will find yourself growing better, and soon after be well.

THE COMPLEAT VERMIN KILLER AND USEFUL POCKET COMPANION, DUBLIN, 1778

POSITIVE CURE FOR AGUE WITHOUT QUININE: Peruvian bark, two ounces; wild cherry-tree bark, one ounce; cinnamon, one dram; capsicum, one teaspoon; sulphur, one ounce; port wine, two quarters; let it stand two days. Buy your Peruvian bark and pulverize it yourself as it is often adulterated otherwise. Dose: one wine glass full every two or three hours after fever is off, then two or three per day till all is used: a certain cure (before taking the above, cleanse the bowels with a dose of epsom salts or other purgative).

DR CASE'S NEW RECIPE BOOK, 1882

Dr Case's claim of a 'positive cure... without quinine' is wrong twice over. Both Peruvian bark and wild cherry bark have quinine properties. Obviously, the great South American cure for ague/malaria was Peruvian bark. However, The People's Home Medical *gives roasted salt the same billing.*

THE GREAT SOUTH AMERICAN REMEDY: Roast some salt in the oven until it is the colour of roasted coffee. Dissolve a soupspoonful in a glass of water and take at one dose. Be careful of the diet.

THE PEOPLE'S HOME MEDICAL BOOK, CLEVELAND, OHIO, 1916

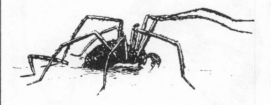

EASY AND ALMOST INSTANTANEOUS CURE FOR AGUE: When the fit is on, take a new laid egg, in a glass of brandy, and go to bed immediately. This very simple remedy has cured a great many after more celebrated preparations have proved unsuccessful.

NEW FAMILY RECEIPT BOOK, LONDON, 1815

How you collect an egg, pour brandy, break the egg into the glass and drink it while shaking from ague is a little difficult to understand. Egg and brandy from one end of the room to the other!

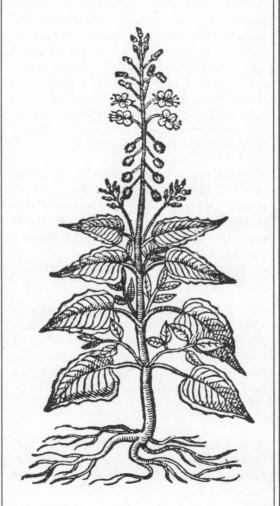

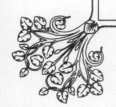
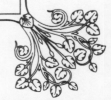

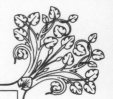

Appetite

To make our appetites more keen,
With eager compounds we our palate urge.
SHAKESPEARE, *SONNET CXVIII*

These eager compounds should start those digestive juices flowing again.

A PLEASANT AND HEALTHY TONIC FOR RESTORING THE APPETITE: Take one ounce pulverized balmony, one ounce pulverized golden seal, one ounce pulverized poplar, half ounce pulverized cloves and put into one quart of good wine (currant or rhubarb is best) with a teacupful of leaf sugar. Let it stand a day or two, shaking it occasionally, and take a wineglassful three times a day, before meals. This is an excellent tonic.
THE HOUSEKEEPER'S GUIDE, OHIO, 1868

TO CREATE AN APPETITE: A piece of rhubarb chewed an hour before dinner is employed by some persons for this purpose. Others such two or three ginger lozenges or take a small glass of bitters.
THE HOUSEHOLD BOOK OF PRACTICAL RECEIPTS, LONDON, 1871

DR. DARWIN'S PILLS FOR WANT OF APPETITE: Take sixty grains of thickened ox-gall, ten grains of conserve of roses. Mix and divide into twelve pills, four of which may be taken half an hour before dinner and supper.
THE FAMILY ORACLE OF HEALTH, ECONOMY, MEDICINE AND GOOD LIVING, LONDON, 1825

The Family Oracle *continued: 'We have remarked that young ladies are often liable to fall into this general disability and we have sometimes ascribed this to their voluntary fasting when they have imagined themselves too plump, and thus they have lost both their health and their beauty, by too great absti-* nence, *often beyond the power of medicine to restore.' Today, we call this phobia about putting on weight anorexia nervosa and have tried to appropriate it as a complaint unique to the 20th century.*

Now, some people, especially sickly youngsters and the elderly, will have very little appetite no matter what you do. For these unfortunates, a snail water was urged to sustain what little strength they had. Just in case you don't have a good recipe for snail water, I have included one.

A SNAIL WATER FOR WEAK CHILDREN AND OLD PEOPLE: Take a pottle of Snails and wash them well in two or three waters and then in small Beer, bruise them shells and all, then put them into a gallon of Red Cow's milk, red rose leaves dried, the whites cut off, Rosemary, marjoram, of each one handful and so distil them in a cold still and let in drop upon powder of white sugar candy in the receiver; drink of it first and last and at four a clock, a wineglass full at a time.
A QUEEN'S DELIGHT, LONDON 1671

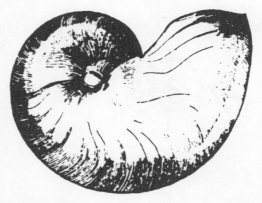

At the other end of the scale are the over-eaters. For them, the world is awash with unfailing cures, miracle diets, guaranteed weight-loss exercises and on and on. Rather than trying to compete in this frenzied war zone, I will just offer this one gentle 16th century remedy.

TO MAKE ONE SLENDER: Take Fennell and seeth it in water, a very good quantity and wringing out the juice thereof when it is sodde, drink it first and last, it will swage either man or woman.
THE GOOD HOUSEWIFE'S JEWELL, THOMAS DAWSON, 1596

If your problem is overeating, you will also find help in the indigestion section.

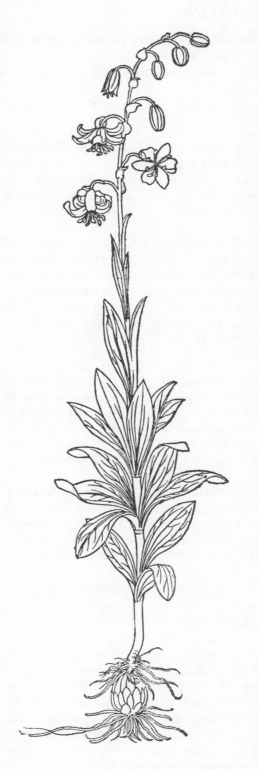

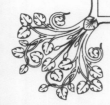
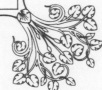

Asthma

You cannot be sure of the success of your remedy, while you are still uncertain of the nature of the disease.

PETER MERE LATHAM (1789–1875)

The nature and causes of asthma still provoke some debate today. So it is no surprise that the suggested remedies for this ailment are diverse, in some cases even in opposition to one another.

A PINT OF COLD WATER every morning and wash the head in cold water and using the cold bath once in two weeks: Or a decoction of liquorice often gives relief; Or half pint of tar water twice a day; Or, live a fortnight chiefly on boiled carrots. It seldom fails.

REVEREND JOHN WESLEY, *PRIMITIVE PHYSICK*, 1747

Reverend John Wesley (1703–91) founder of the Methodist Church, wrote a book of simple cures for his followers. The pocket-sized manual was published in 1747 as Primitive Physick: *or* An Easy and Natural Way of Curing Most Diseases.

IN ASTHMA, it is a great relief to place the feet, knees and elbows pretty deep in warm water. The patient should be carefully guarded from taking cold.

LYDIA CHILD, *THE FAMILY NURSE*, BOSTON, 1837

Choose your own medicine—cold baths or a warm soak. Either is far easier to live with than the Tennessee remedy which insists that asthma can be cured by rendering down the scent glands of a pole cat (skunk) and rubbing it on the chest of the patient. If that's too pungent, for less intensity but the same essence try skunk cabbage.

TAKE THE ROOTS OF SKUNK CABBAGE, dry and pulverize them and give three doses per day until cured. Give at a dose what will lay on the end of a pen knife.

JOHN STONER'S SYMPATHY—A COLLECTION OF EXCELLENT REMEDIES AND RECIPES FOR THE CURE OF VARIOUS DISEASES OF PERSONS AND CATTLE, OHIO 1867

TEXAS REMEDIES:

• Get a Mexican hairless (chihuahua) dog and keep it nearby. The asthma will go from you to the dog. You can not use someone else's dog.

• Sleep in sand pits containing small amounts of uranium. Get a muskrat skin and wear it over your lungs with the fur side next to the body.

• Sleep on the wool of a sheep that has recently been clipped. Do not clean or wash the wool. The asthma will be absorbed into the wool.

• String a line of crickets on a silk string and wear them crickets around the neck.

If you prefer amber to crickets, a Kentucky remedy claims you may cure asthma by wearing a string of amber beads around the neck.

Contradiction continued to be the rule in asthma remedies. Even the great English herbalist, Nicholas Culpeper (1616–54) had his advice disputed. The U.S. Practical Receipt Book noted in 1844 that for a dry or convulsive Asthma, 'it is said that the juice of radishes is good in this complaint.' In contrast, Culpeper was contemptuous of the curative properties of the lowly radish. He said, 'Garden Raddishes are in wantoness by the gentry eaten as a sallad, but they breed scurvy humours in the stomach and corrupt

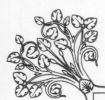

the blood and then send for a physician as fast as you can.' Culpeper was far more enthusiastic about horehound. He endorsed it in The English Physician, *in which he noted,*

THERE IS A SYRUP, made of horehound, to be had at the apothecaries, very good for old coughs, to rid phlegm; as also to avoid cold rheum from the lungs of old folks, and for those who are asthmatic or short-winded.

Dr Chase actually agreed that horehound would relieve asthma.

ELECAMPANE, ANGELICA, COMFREY, and spikenard roots, with hoarhound tops, of each one ounce. Bruise and steep in honey, one pint. Dose: a tablespoon taken hot every few minutes until relief is obtained, then several times daily until a cure is effected.
DR CHASE'S RECIPES, 1867 EDITION

For those who prefer to take their medicine in the privacy of their own bedroom, here are a few suggestions to relieve the wheezing.

ASTHMA HAS BEEN CURED by sleeping on a pillow made of wild balsam, or, as many people call it, life everlasting. The remedy is so simple that it deserves a trial.
THE HEARTHSTONE, PHILADELPHIA 1883

TO RELIEVE ASTHMA, make a pad of five layers of strong unbleached calico, wring out of cold water, and place it on the sufferer's chest, keep it wet. This has been known to cure very obstinate cases.
THE AUSTRALIAN HOUSEHOLD MANUAL, 1899

DIP A BROWN PAPER the size of two hands in strong saltpetre water and burn the same in the room before going to bed. It will give great relief.
FARMER'S DIRECTORY AND HOUSEKEEPER'S ASSISTANT, TORONTO, 1851

This last cure was used by the Indians throughout many regions of the Americas. If it does not help your asthma, you probably won't care anyway. Stramonium, also known as Jimson weed or thornapple, can be lethal if taken in large doses. However, smoked in small doses, stramonium, as the Indians discovered, is a relaxant and hallucinogen.

A CURE FOR ASTHMA: Take the stalk of stramonium three inches above the ground, and the root connected with it: dry it and pulverize it. When the asthmatic paroxysms take place, smoke it as much you would tobacco and as much of it as you can bear: when the paroxysms are over, smoke it two or three times everyday. This course pursued will effect a final cure.
THE FAMILY PHYSICIAN AND THE FARMER'S COMPANION, SYRACUSE, NEW YORK, 1840

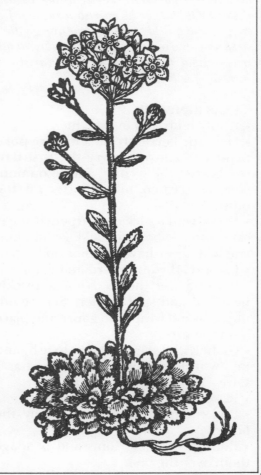

Boils

Thou art a boil,
A Plague sore, an embossed carbuncle
In my corrupted blood.
SHAKESPEARE, *KING LEAR*

The Bible was often the only book our ances-tors owned. As well as being a source of inspiration, it was also a source of advice. Isaiah 38:21 was commonly quoted as a cure for boils. This verse urges: 'Let them take a lump of figs and lay it for a plaster upon the boil and he shall recover.' Herbalist Nicholas Culpeper attributed the fig tree with magical powers: 'They say that the fig tree, as well as the bay tree, is never hurt by lightning, as also if you tie a bull, be he ever so mad, to a fig tree, he will quickly become tame and gentle.'

If you are out of figs, take heart, those irrepressible Texans had quite a variety of remedies for boils:

TEXAS REMEDIES:
• Apply fat bacon overnight.
• Pick ripe berries from a mature poke plant and eat one berry the first day, two berries the second, and so on until you have eaten nine berries on the ninth day.
• Pierce with a stick of sharpened sugar cane and the boil will heal. In addition you will never have another boil.
• Fry a road runner bird and eat it.
• Remove the thorns from a prickly pear leaf and split it open. Scrape out the pulp and wrap it on gauze and place it on the sore.
• Gather wild daisies, burn to ash, and mix with lard. This is to be used as a salve.
• Place hot cow manure on boils.
• Boil mesquite beans and apply the liquid.
• Boil up okra blossoms and bandage them over the boil.

FOR SUPPURATION OF MAN OR BEAST: Take a field toad which, during harvest time, has been put upon a stick and placed in a position toward the rising sun where it died. Of such a toad take the corresponding limb of that part of which the patient suffers, be it man or beast, and tie it to the ailing limb.
ALBERTUS MAGNUS OR EGYPTIAN SECRETS

The Australian Kandy Koola Cook Book *describes the following treatment for a boil. A druggist in an apothecary museum also rec-ommended it to me as a safe and amazingly rapid cure.*

THE SKIN OF A BOILED EGG is the best remedy for a boil. Carefully peel it, wet, and apply to the boil. It draws out mat-ter and relieves soreness.

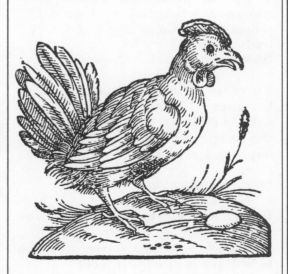

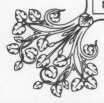
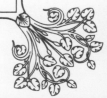

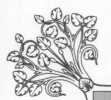

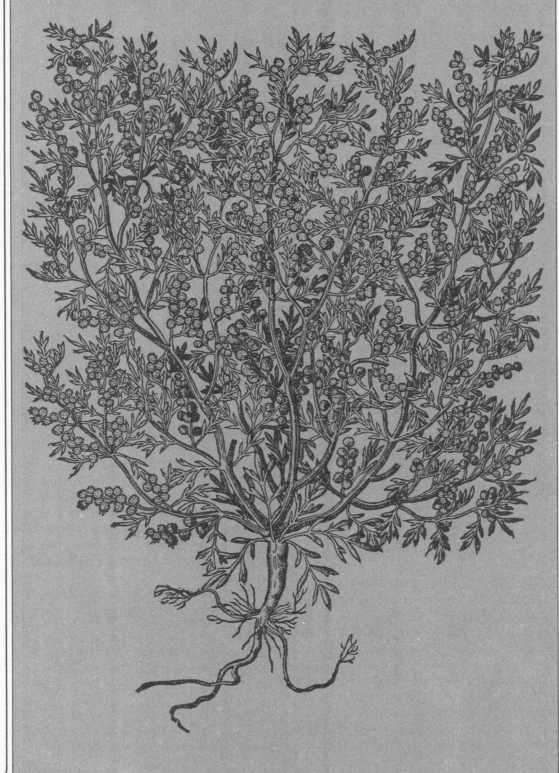

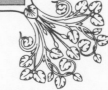

Cankers

Until the 17th century, the word canker *was used to mean what we now call cancer. But over time, the word evolved to its more specialized meaning, namely those hateful little ulcerated sores which cause so much pain on the gums and tongue.*

This first remedy begins pleasantly enough...

A CURE FOR THE CANKER IN THE MOUTH AND THROAT: Take one pound of fresh butter, put it into an earthen vessel well glazed, sit it to the fire, let it boil, when boiling add to it four common green frogs, put them in alive, let them stew until they are dry, take them out, add to it a little camomile and parsley; when cold, stir in a little burnt alum. This will cure the most inveterate canker in the mouth, throat or stomach.
THE FAMILY PHYSICIAN AND FARMER'S COMPANION, SYRACUSE, NEW YORK, 1840.

The North American Indians made common use of all the ingredients in the following recipe. In fact, gold thread also goes by the name canker root and was chewed by the Indians for mouth sores.

THIS IS AN ACRID HUMOUR excoriating the most tender parts, particularily the mouth. Frequent applications of the decoction of cranesbill, wild lettuce, white lilly, or gold thread affords relief.
U.S. PRACTICAL RECEIPT BOOK 1844

If you do not have the above ingredients readily available, perhaps you will have better luck with these:

THE COMMON DARK BLUE VIOLET makes a slimy tea, which is excellent for a canker. Leaves and blossoms are both good.
LYDIA CHILD, *THE FRUGAL HOUSEWIFE,* BOSTON, 1831

Lydia Maria Child was an enlightened abolitionist who was not afraid to go against public opinion and speak out against slavery to the Boston establishment in the 1830s. However, she was less bold when writing of hygiene and health matters, as she explained in the foreword to The Family Nurse or Companion of the Frugal Housewife *in 1837. 'This volume is very obviously not intended for the drawing room. If written in language plain enough to be understood, it could not be in the very nature of the subject, be otherwise than indelicate, in the world's esteem. Considerations of this kind induced me to lay it aside for a long time unfinished.'*

BURN A CORN COB and apply the ashes two or three times a day.
CANADIAN PIONEER REMEDY

THE BEST TREATMENT for this painful malady is to gargle the mouth and throat with a wash prepared by steeping red raspberry leaves in water. A little sugar may be added to soften the astringent power of the decoction.
FARMER'S DIRECTORY AND HOUSEKEEPER'S ASSISTANT, TORONTO, 1851

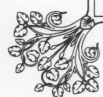
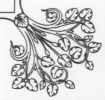

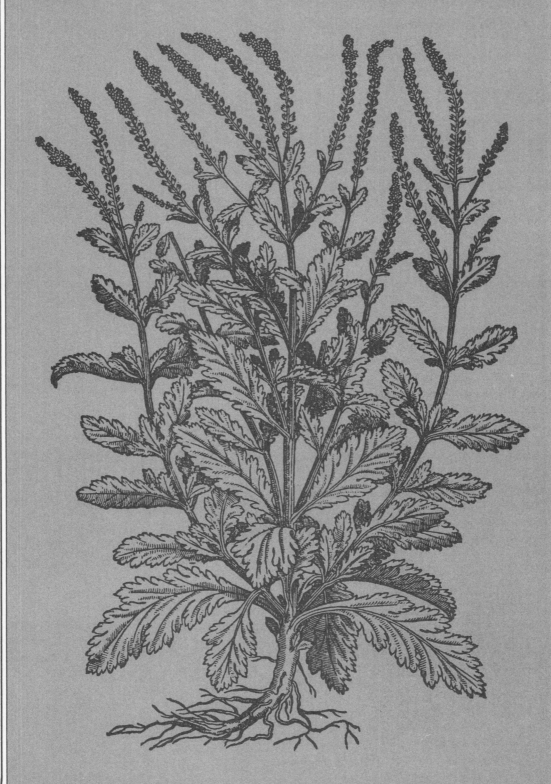

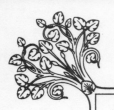

Chilblains

Another weepeth over chilblains fell,
Always upon the heel yet never to be well.
THOMAS HOOD (1799-1845) *THE IRISH*
SCHOOLMASTER

Most young people today have never heard of chilblains. However, they could make a comeback because of the renewed popularity of potbelly stoves and fireplaces. Chilblains describe painful swellings of the hands and feet, in which the skin turns a leaden or purple colour accompanied by irritation, itching, tenderness and shooting pains. And the most common cause is holding the hands and feet to the fire immediately after they have been exposed to the cold. Country people believed the acid in urine was the best cure and bathed their hands and feet in the contents of their chamber pots. Since I hope the chamber pot will not be making a similar comeback, I have included a few other remedies.

CHILBLAINS: TO CURE—PUBLISHED BY ORDER OF THE GOVERNMENT OF WIRTENBERG: Mutton tallow and lard, of each ¾ of a pound; melt in an iron vessel and add hydrated oxyde of iron, two ounces; stirring continually with an iron spoon, until the mass is of an uniform black colour; then let it cool and add venice turpentine, two ounces; and armenian bole, one ounce; oil of bergamot, one dram; rub up the bole with a little olive oil before putting it in. Apply several times daily, by putting it upon lint or linen—heals the worst cases in a few days.
DR CHASE'S RECIPES, 1867 EDITION

THE THIN SKIN that comes from suet is good to bind upon the feet for chilblains. Rubbing them with spirits of turpentine, or castille soap and honey, frequently and perseveringly is much recommended. A wash made of chamomile flowers and poppy seedvessels is useful; to be followed by the application of cooling ointments. Sometimes it becomes necessary to apply leeches to chilblains and take active physic.
LYDIA CHILD, *THE FAMILY NURSE,* BOSTON, 1837

Another expression for chilblains is kibed heel. The following use very simple ingredients found in most kitchens.

A POULTICE FOR KIBED HEELS: Take onions and turnips roasted, of each what pleases, mix with turpentine, what suffices; for kibed heels.
THE FAMILY MAGAZINE, LONDON 1741.

TAKE PRETTY THICK PARINGS fresh cut from turnips, and hold them to the fire till crisp; then apply them to the unbroken tumours or blisters, as hot as can be endured and keep them on a competent time, and repeat them, if requir'd. They will relieve without breaking the blisters.
THE FAMILY MAGAZINE, LONDON 1741.

Finally, Reverend Wesley gives advice on how to prevent getting chilblains in the first place.

WEAR FLANNEL SOCK, or socks of chamois leather.
REVEREND JOHN WESLEY, *PRIMITIVE PHYSICK,* 1747.

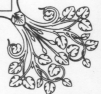

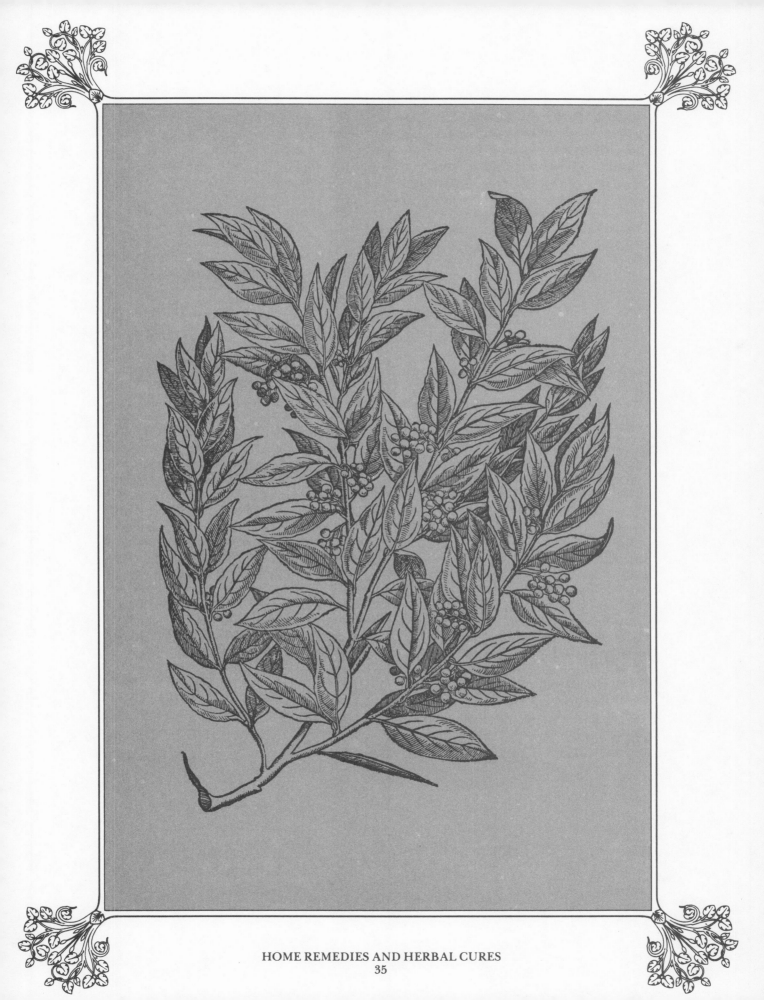

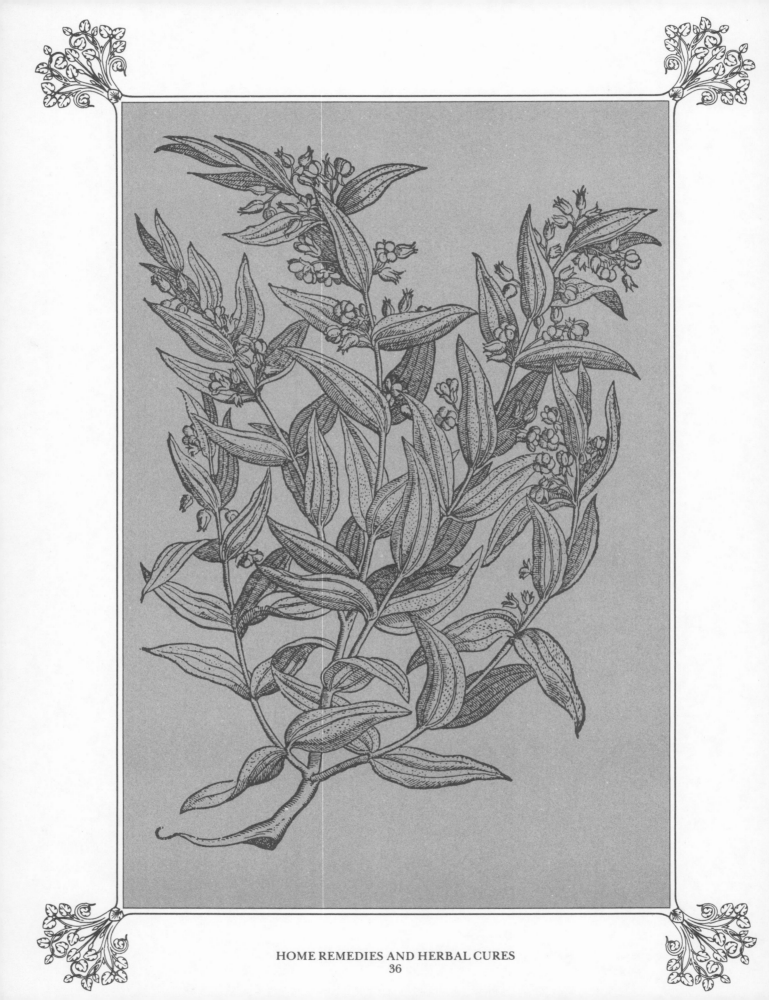

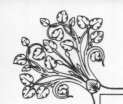

Colds and Coughs

Ye can call it influenza if ye like, said Mrs. Machin. There was no influenza in my young days. We call a cold a cold.
ARNOLD BENNETT, *THE CARD*

COLDS: This must be strictly attended to every evening, that is, whenever you pull off your shoes or stockings, run your finger between all the toes and smell it. This will certainly effect a cure.
THE LONG LOST FRIEND, 1856.

The Long Lost Friend *also recommends the toe-sniff cure as a remedy for hysterics! John George Hohman was the reluctant author of this little book first published in 1820. He told his readers that he really had not wanted to publish it and his wife was also opposed to the idea. However, his compassion for the suffering of his fellow men had compelled him to share his knowledge. 'Besides,' he said, 'I'm a poor man in needy circumstances, and it is a little help to me if I can make a little money with the sale of my books.'*

COLD IN THE HEAD: M. Farn, a Belgian physician, says a cold may often be arrested by a brisk friction of the back of the head with some stimulating lotion, as lavender water, sal-volatile etc. Also a similar rubbing two or three times a week will prevent the 'catching' of a cold by those who are liable to do so from slight causes.
DR CHASE'S RECIPES, 1880 EDITION

Here are some very early English cold remedies. In the 10th and 11th centuries, the monks were the main source of medical knowledge and kept elaborate physic gardens to provide the medicinal herbs and plants. Later, the Lady of the Manor took over these duties, spending much of her time in her garden or still-room concocting potions from the family recipe book. Ann Blencowe, wife of John, member of Parliament for Brackley, Northamptonshire from 1690 to 1695, tended her household while her husband tended to Parliament.

FOR A COLD IN YE HEAD: Take sage leaves, rub them and apply them to ye nostrils in the morning.
THE RECEIPT BOOK OF MRS. ANN BLENCOWE 1694.

Nicholas Culpeper recommended sage to help the memory and quicken the senses. He didn't say how you should deal with people joking about the sage on your nose!

FOR TIGHT CHEST: Boil holly bark in goat's milk and sip warm, fasting.
LACNUNGA, EARLY ANGLO-SAXON REMEDY

FOR A COLD: Take a quarter of a pint of horehound water, a quarter of a pint of coltsfoot water, a pound of reasons (raisins) of the sun stoned, pound the reasons very well then mingle these together then set them on the fire boyle them like marmolet then take it off and put it into two ounces of honey and one spoonfull mustard then set it on the fire and let it simmer a while then put it into a pot and take as much as ye quantity of a walnut first in ye morning and last at night.
A BOOK OF SIMPLES, LONDON, 1750.

MRS. HELEN PARRY'S RECEIPTE FOR A COLD: Take ye fairest orange you can get rost it at ye fire then put thereto a pretty quantity of sallet oyle sweeten it with sugar candie or sugar drinking it 1st in ye morning and last at night.
A BOOK OF SIMPLES, LONDON, 1750

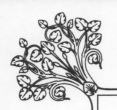

A May cold is a thirty day cold.
ENGLISH PROVERB

George Washington may have taken the credit for the next remedy, but in Europe, peasants had already been using it for centuries. Other favourites were a syrup of onions and sugar or raw onions chopped fine, sprinkled with gum camphor, placed in a flannel and laid on the chest. In Kentucky, to keep off a cold the people would cut an onion in half, hang it by a string and knock it every time they passed. It was widely believed that onions absorbed germs and it was common practice to place a saucer of sliced onions under a sickbed to attract the germs.

GENERAL WASHINGTON'S COLD CURE: The Baltimore American informs us that General George Washington gave the following recipe for a cold to an old lady now living in Newport when she was a very young girl (1781). He was lodging in her father's house, the old Vermont mansion. As she was being sent to bed early with a very bad cold he remarked to Mrs Vernon, the mother of this lady: 'My own remedy, my dear Madam, is always to eat, just before I step into bed, a hot roasted onion, if I have a cold.'
DR. CHASE'S RECIPES, 1892 EDITION

HERE'S A GOOD TIP for anyone eating raw onions: chewing a piece of apple, parsley, a raw green bean, a little aniseed, or coffee beans gets rid of onion breath.

People tend to find use for resources at hand. Texans seem to have found many uses for the ever-present supply of cow manure. And the Australians have evolved many recipes using eucalyptus oil.

TEXAS REMEDIES:
• Apply fresh cow dung to your chest in the form of a cross.
• Wear the skin of a white weasel around your neck.
• Rub the bottom of your feet with tallow and turpentine. and then hold your feet against an old wood stove.
• Put some mequite leaves under your hat.
• Rub the chest with goose grease and kerosene.
• Catching leaves in your hand which fall from the trees in the Fall will cure a head cold.
• Take dried frog skins and make a powder of them. Mix with fruit juice and drink.

AUSTRALIAN REMEDY: Extract of eucalyptus is valuable for coughs and colds, but should be used sparingly if taken internally, as overdoses have very injurious effects. For cold in the head, moisten the nostrils with the spirit frequently.
THE AUSTRALIAN HOUSEHOLD MANUAL, 1899

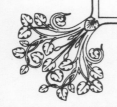
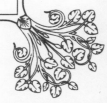

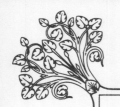

'Tis dangerous to take a cold.
SHAKESPEARE, *HENRY IV*

We now turn to the heavy-duty remedies. If you try the first one, see the headache section for a hangover cure.

A WESTERN RANCHER SUGGESTS THIS CURE FOR A BAD COLD: Put your hat on the table, drink well from a bottle of good whiskey until you see two hats. Then get into bed and stay there.
CANADIAN PRAIRIES REMEDY

COLD; One tablespoon molasses, two teaspoons castor oil, one teaspoon paregoric, one teaspoon spirits camphor. Mix them and take it often. Will cure any cold.
RECIPE IN CANADIAN PIONEER'S DOCTOR-BOOK, QUOTED IN *AN HISTORICAL ALMANAC OF CANADA*

If the last remedy did not cure your cold, you probably would not even care, because paregoric is camphorated tincture of opium. Opium was the aspirin of the 19th century and was used for many of the same complaints: hangovers, pain and fatigue. It was given to babies in liberal doses to keep them quiet and soothed. Dr Chase gave his readers a recipe for paregoric:

Best opium, one drachm, dissolve in about two tablespoons of boiling water; then add benzoic acid, half drachm; oil of anise, half a fluid drachm; clarified honey, one oz.; camphor gum, one scruple ($^{1}/_{24}$th of an ounce); alcohol (76%), eleven fluid ounces, distilled water, four and a half fluid oz. Steep (keep warm) for two weeks. Dose: for children five to twenty drops. Adults: one or two teaspoons.

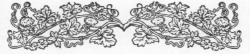

Dr Chase's prescription in the next remedy is the opposite of that old English saying 'stuff a cold and starve a fever.'

LET A MAN EAT NEXT TO NOTHING for two days, providing he is not confined to bed, for by taking no carbon into the system by food and by consuming the surplus which caused his disease, by breath, he soon carries off his disease by removing the cause. This will be found more effectual if he adds copious water draughts to the protracted fasting. By the time a person has fasted one day and night, he will experience a freedom from disease and a clearness of mind, in a delightful contrast with mental stupor and physical pain caused by colds.
DR CHASE'S RECIPES, 1880 EDITION

Reverend Wesley gave doses of advice along with his cures. Here's one of his plain easy rules for keeping healthy: 'nothing conduces more health than abstinence and plain food, with due labour.' And if you still get a cold, he suggests the following.

A COLD: Drink a pint of cold water lying down in bed (tried)
OR to one spoonful of molasses in half a pint of water (tried) or, to one spoonful of oatmeal, and one spoonful of honey, add a piece of butter the bigness of a nutmeg; pour on gradually near a pint of boiling water. Drink this lying down in bed.
OR
A COLD IN THE HEAD: Pare very thin the yellow rind of an orange, roll it up inside out and thrust a roll into each nostril.
REVEREND JOHN WESLEY, *PRIMITIVE PHYSICK*, 1747

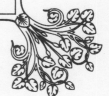

COUGH: A convulsion of the lungs vellicated by some sharp serosity.
FROM SAMUEL JOHNSON'S *DICTIONARY*, 1755.

More common English folk than Samuel Johnson believed in the magical transfer of disease from people to plants and animals. You will find many other examples of magical transference in this book, especially in the warts section. Dogs seem to be the poor victims in many cases. For example, a Texas remedy for asthma suggests buying a chihuahua dog and keeping it near the asthma victim. The asthma is supposed to shift into the dog.

CURE FOR A COUGH: Put the hair of the patient's head between two slices of buttered bread and give the sandwich to a dog. The animal will therefore catch the cough and the patient will lose it.
A NORTHAMPTONSHIRE, DEVONSHIRE AND WELSH FOLK REMEDY

When the next remedy first appeared in The Farmer's Advocate *in October 1876, it called for half a cup of ginger instead of vinegar. The next edition of the paper made the correction and neither version gave the dosage. The correction was probably made when a reader complained; that is, when he could talk again.*

COUGH AND SORE THROAT: Take one cup honey, half cup vinegar, one small teaspoonful cayenne pepper.
THE FARMER'S ADVOCATE, LONDON, ONTARIO, OCTOBER 1876

FOR A VIOLENT COUGH ARISING FROM AN ASTHMA: Infuse three drachms of garlick and half an ounce of mustard seed into a quart of white wine, let it stand a week closed up and drink a glass of it as often as you please.
THE COMPLEAT VERMIN KILLER AND USEFUL POCKET COMPANION, DUBLIN, 1778

If you prefer a sweeter-tasting medicine, take a look at these.

THREE NEWLY LAID EGGS, unbroken, over which pour the juice of six lemons and allow to stand for forty-eight hours. Then pick out any bits of egg shell which are not dissolved. Add one half pound of rock candy and one pint of Jamaica brandy: mix well and bottle. Dose: one tablespoon three or four times a day.
THE NEW COOK BOOK, TORONTO, 1906

A CONSUMPTIVE COUGH: To stop it for a time, at lying down keep a little stick liquorice shaved like horseradish between the cheek and gums. I believe this never fails.
OR
A CONVULSIVE COUGH: Eat preserved walnuts.
OR
A TICKLING COUGH: Drink water whitened with oatmeal four times a day.
Or, keep a piece of barley sugar or sugar candy constantly in the mouth.
REVEREND JOHN WESLEY, *THE PRIMITIVE PHYSICK*, 1747

THE HONOURABLE MR. BOYLE'S GENUINE SIRUP FOR COUGHS: This excellent remedy cannot be made too public. It is thus prepared. Take six ounces of cumfrey root and twelve handfuls of plantain leaves: cut and beat them well: strain out the juice: and with an equal weight of sugar, boil it to a sirup.
UNIVERSAL RECEIPT BOOK CONTAINING SCARCE, CURIOUS AND VALUABLE RECEIPTS AND CHOICE SECRETS BY A SOCIETY OF GENTLEMEN IN NEW YORK, 1814

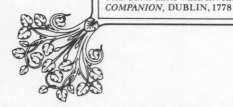
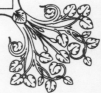

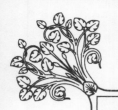

Love and a cough cannot be hidden.

AN EASY MEDICINE FOR A DRY HUSKING COUGH: Drink near a pint of spring water, as hot as you can, the last thing you do, going to rest. This is recommended by one whose integrity may be depended on, and tho' 'tis seemingly a trifling prescription, it has done very wonderful cures.
A COLLECTION OF RECEIPTS IN COOKERY PHYSICK AND SURGERY, LONDON, 1749

This book was written by Mrs Mary Kettilby 'for the use of Good Wives, Tender Mothers and Careful Nurses.'

COUGHS: If you dry chestnuts (only the kernels I mean) both the barks being taken away, beat them into powder and make the powder up into an electuary with honey, so you have an admirable remedy for the cough and spitting of blood.
NICHOLAS CULPEPER, *THE ENGLISH PHYSICIAN,* 1652

The next couple of cures come from the diary of a Canadian pioneer. Valued remedies were copied or clipped out of newspapers and passed down to the next generation. And just as the Australian settlers learned of the medicinal value of goanna fat and eucalyptus from the Aborigines, so did the North American pioneers take heed of native medicines. All these ingredients were used by the Indians for a variety of complaints. White oak bark was used as a substitute for quinine; slippery elm as a poultice or a brew for stomach disorders and coughs and colds.

SLIPPERY ELM COUGH CURE: Break the bark into little bits, pour boiling water on it until covered, then cover the dish and leave it until it is cold. Sweeten and take for summer disorders or add lemon juice and drink for bad colds.

EXCELLENT COUGH CURE: Buttonwood, white oak and white ash barks, equal parts boiled in water and sweetened with honey. Dose: one tablespoon three times a day.

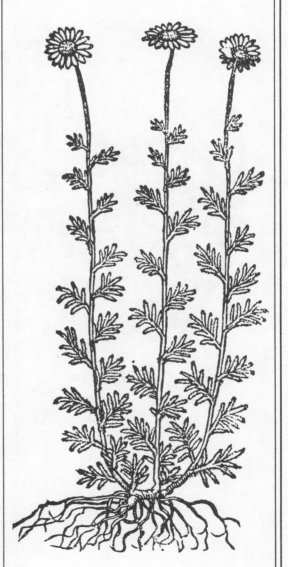

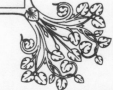
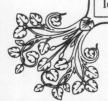

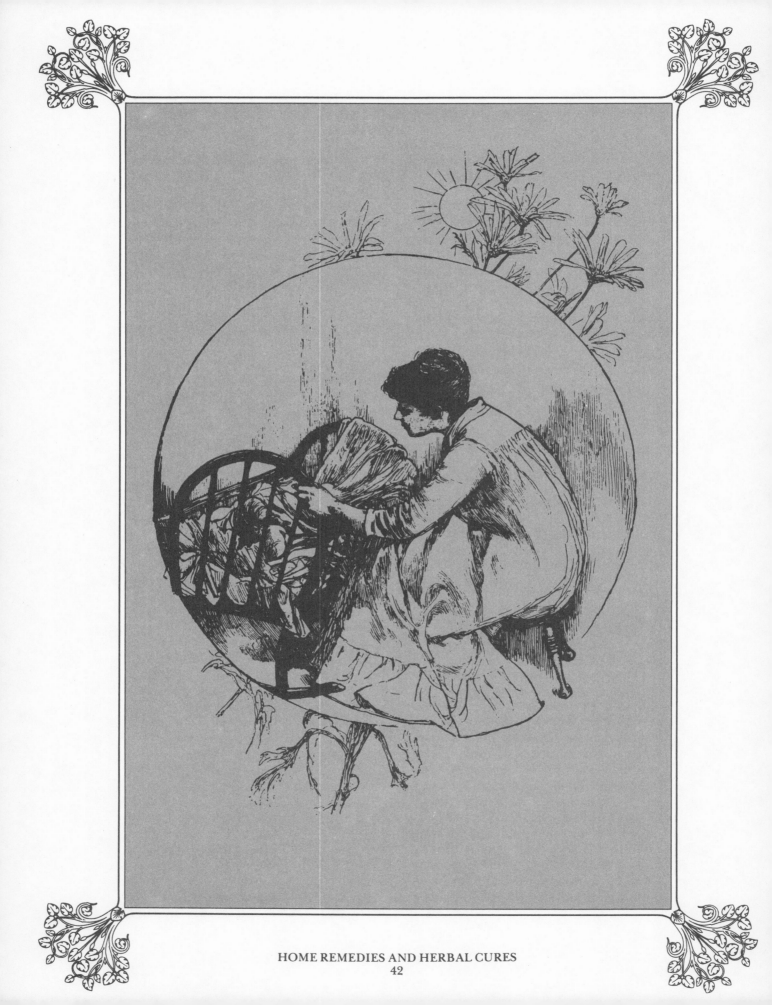

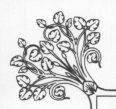

Colic

Oft the teeming earth
Is with a kind of colic pinch'd and vex'd
By the imprisoning of unruly wind
  within her womb.
SHAKESPEARE, *HENRY IV*

Although colic is usually associated with unhappy babies, adults too can suffer from these spasmodic stomach pains. Here's how the Texans soothed their babies.

TEXAS REMEDIES:
• Close the windows and doors of the baby's room and have someone smoke and keep smoking with a pipe or cigar.
• Give the baby mare's milk in small doses.
• Give the child one teaspoonful of water that has passed through a chimney ash or soot filter. Give this before every feeding.

The next two remedies came from a manuscript of cookery and medical recipes in Samuel Pepys' library. This manuscript of miscellaneous recipes was probably compiled during the last years of the 15th century, during the reign of Henry VII.

FOR THE COLIC AND THE STONE: Take lettuce, viperal, cinquefoil, hissop, dragonwort, hartstongue, violets, dandelion, equal quantities of each and boil with a cock of a red colour.
STERE ITT WELL

Incidentally, cinquefoil was believed to be a standard ingredient in witches' ointment and was also hung in doorways to keep out evil spirits.

A GOOD MEDICINE FOR THE COLIC: Take the hulls of green beans and distil them and make water thereof and use that fasting with a little stale ale until you are eased thereof.
STERE ITT WELL

Although Pepys had catalogued this manuscript himself, an entry in his diary dated 26 March 1655 would lead us to believe he had rejected these remedies himself for something simpler. 'Now I am at a loss to know whether it be my hare's foot which is my preservation; for I never had a fit of collique since I wore it, or whether it be my taking of a pill of turpentine every morning.'

Punch cures the gout, the colic, and the 'tisick
And is by all agreed the very best of physic.
ENGLISH RHYME (18TH C.)

The next remedies certainly took the advice contained in the rhyme.

A VERY GOOD REMEDY FOR THE COLIC: Take half a gill of good rye whiskey, and a pipe full of tobacco; put the whiskey in a bottle, then smoke the tobacco and blow the smoke into the bottle, shake it up and drink it. This has cured the author of this book and many others. Or take a white clay pipe which has turned blackish from smoking, pound it to a fine powder and take it. This will have the same effect.
THE LONG LOST FRIEND, 1856

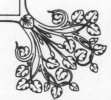

TINCTURE OF RHUBARB, EXCELLENT IN THE COLICK: Take rhubarb sliced thin, two ounces; brandy, one quart; infuse cold. For some uses 'tis best to infuse it in cinnamon water. The dose: Three or four ounces.
THE FAMILY MAGAZINE, LONDON, 1741

FOR THE BILIOUS COLIC: West India rum, one gill; West India molasses, one gill; hog's lard, one gill; and the urine of a beast, one gill; simmer them together, take one gill every half hour; I have never known this to fail.
FAMILY PHYSICIAN AND THE FARMER'S COMPANION,
SYRACUSE, NEW YORK, 1840

Take a few bay leaves and soak them in brandy in a warm room. As soon as the colic is felt, take from one to four spoonfuls of this remedy.
ALBERTUS MAGNUS OR EGYPTIAN SECRETS

A GERMAN REMEDY OR LINIMENT FOR COLIC: Alcohol, one quart; oil of sassafras and hartshorn, each two ounces; spirits of camphor and laudanum, each one ounce; spirits of turpentine, half an ounce; tincture of kino, one-quarter ounce; mix. Dose: for colic, or any severe internal pain, from half to one teaspoonful may be taken for a dose, to be repeated in half to one hour according to the severity of the case.
DR CHASE'S RECIPES, 1892 EDITION

Dr Chase gave his readers a recipe for making laudanum. 'Best Turkey Opium, one ounce, slice and pour upon it boiling water, one gill and work it in a bowl or mortar until it is dissolved; then pour it into the bottle and with alcohol of 76% proof, half a pint, rinse the dish adding the alcohol to the preparation, shaking well and in twenty-four hours it will be ready for use. Dose: from ten to thirty drops for adults according to the strength of the patient or severity of the pain. Thirty drops of this laudanum will equal to one grain of opium.' Like paregoric, laudanum was used for a variety of complaints.

Laudanum gave me repose, not sleep:
but you, I believe, know how divine
this repose is, what a spot of enchantment,
a green spot of fountain and flowers
and trees in the very heart of a waste
of sand.
SAMUEL COLERIDGE, (1772–1834)

Every mother knows the curative powers of a nourishing bowl of chicken broth and Ann Blencowe was no exception in 1694. She may have been a little excessive in the quantity.

GOOD IN A FITT OF YE COLICK: To take a great Quantity of chicken broth, a gallon or more.
THE RECEIPT BOOK OF MRS. ANN BLENCOWE, 1694

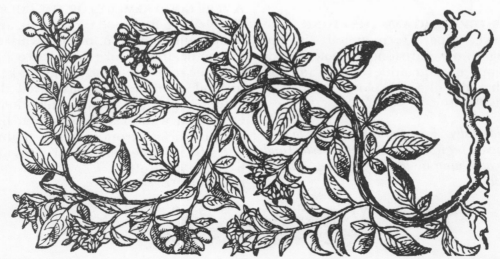

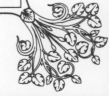

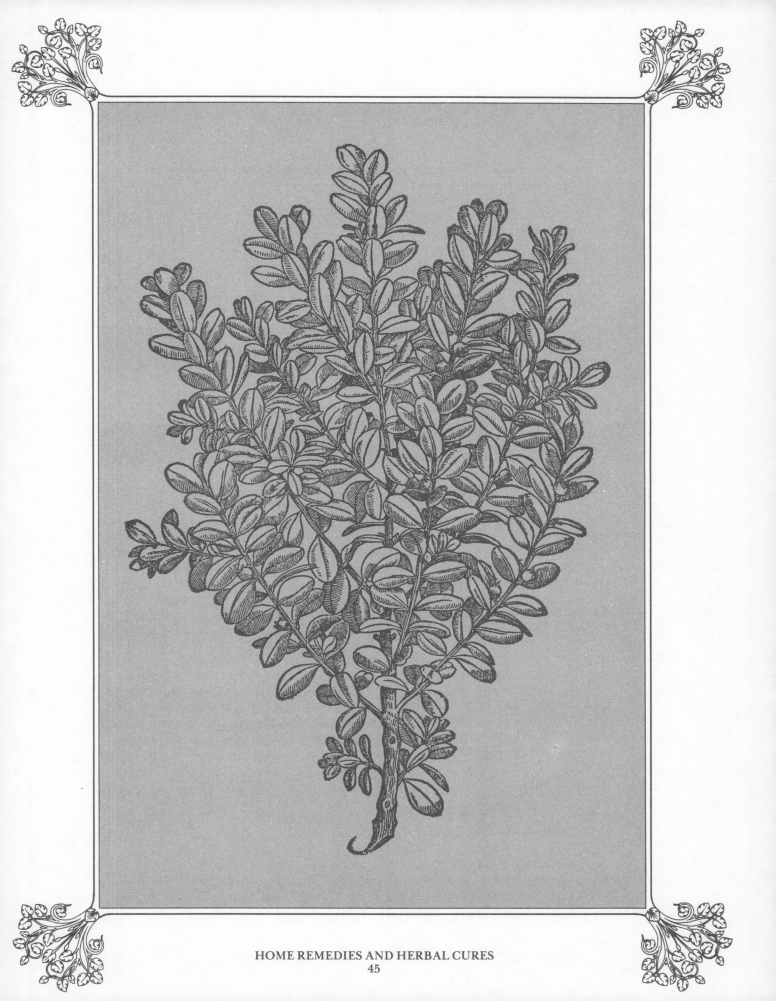

Constipation

I have finally kum to the konklusion that a reliable sett ov bowels iz worth more tu a man, than enny quantity ov brains.

JOSH BILLINGS, *HIS SAYINGS*

Our ancestors probably did not suffer as much from constipation because they were not tempted with all the refined foods we find on grocery shelves today. But since they also could not reach out for prepared laxatives, they all had family favourites for this complaint. The simplest and most economical remedy for constipation is a cup of hot water, which can be sweetened with a teaspoonful of honey and usually taken before breakfast.

Mrs Gorman from Dickson, Australia, sent me this remedy which she got from her 87-year-old father, who in turn remembers the recipe from his mother's preparation. Like Christmas cake, the ingredients have sky-rocketed in price!

HALF A POUND OF RAISINS, half a pound of dates, half a pound of figs, two ounces powdered senna, one ounce powdered sulphur and half an ounce of powdered ginger. Mix powdered ingredients together, put all the fruit through the mincer twice, then blend well with the dry ingredients. If too dry, add a teaspoon of glycerine. Take a small portion at bedtime.

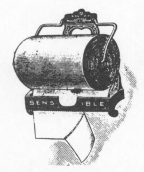

CORNMEAL: One tablespoon of cornmeal stirred up in sufficient cold water to drink well and drank in the morning immediately after rising, has, with perseverance, cured many bad cases.

OR

A FRESH EGG: Beat in a gill of water and drank on rising in the morning and at each meal for a week to ten days, has cured obstinate cases. It might be increased to two or three at a time as the stomach will bear.

OR

BRANDY, half a pint; and put into it rhubarb-root, bruised, one drachm, hiera-picra, one ounce; and fennel seed, half an ounce. After it has stood for several days, take a tablespoon for it three times daily, before eating until it operates, then half the quantity, or a little less, just sufficient to establish a daily action of the bowels until all is taken.

DR CHASE'S RECIPES, 1867 EDITION

Hiera-picra is commonly known as "hickory-pickory". It is a powder composed of aloes and canella which is used both as a laxative and as an agent to promote menstruation.

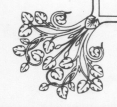
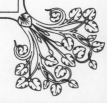

Reverend Wesley had a simple solution for constipation. He urged: 'Rise early every morning.' But if this failed, the good cleric had backups.

BOIL IN A PINT AND A HALF OF BROTH, half a handful of mallow leaves chopped, strain this and drink it before you eat anything else. Do this frequently, if needful.

OR, take the bigness of a large nutmeg of cream of tartar mixed with honey, as often as you need.

OR, take daily, two hours before dinner a small teacupful of stewed prunes.

OR, boil an ounce and a half tamarinds in three pints of water to a quart. In this, strained, when cold, infuse all night two drachms of senna, and one drachm of red rose leaves, drink a cupful every morning.

REVEREND JOHN WESLEY, *PRIMITIVE PHYSICK,* 1747

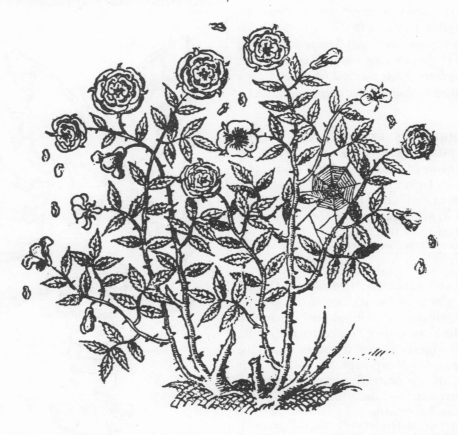

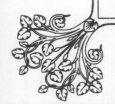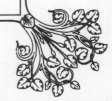

Consumption

It was all the fashion to suffer from chest complaint; everyone was consumptive, poets especially; it was good form to spit blood after each emotion that was at all inclined to be sensational, and to die before reaching thirty.

ALEXANDRE DUMAS (1802–70)

Consumption, or tuberculosis as it is known today, has been with man from earliest times. It went by several names, the more common being maramus, literally meaning wasting away, phthisis, scrofula and king's evil. It got that last name from the superstition that royalty could cure the disease by a touch of the hand. As Alexandre Dumas rather cynically observed, a disproportionate number of victims were artists.

I have included this section to illustrate one of the success stories of modern medicine. Although, unlike smallpox, consumption has not been eradicated, this highly contagious bacterial disease can now be treated with great success. That was not likely with these misguided and often nasty cures below.

DR GIBBONS'S RECEIPT FOR A CONSUMPTION INSTEAD OF ASSES MILK: To three pints of water put forty snails, two ounces of eringo roots, two ounces of french brandy; boil it to one quart, then strain it, and take two spoonfuls in half a pint of milk twice a day.

THE ACCOMPLISHED HOUSEWIFE—RECEIPTS IN PHYSICK, 1754

TAKE AN OLD COCK, a beast's foot, four ounces of goatshorn shaving, six poppy heads, cinnamon, cloves and nutmegs, each half an ounce, mace, two drams; boil all together until it comes to a jelly, add as much lump sugar as will make it sweet, after it is strained add a bottle of red port wine—take a teacup full every night and morning.

MRS BENJAMIN SMITH, NEWFOUNDLAND (FROM HER FAMILY'S DOCTOR BOOK), 1841

A NOURISHING MEDICINE FOR CONSUMPTIVE LADIES: Take a dozen of crayfish of the smallest sort, gut them clean, and let them be boiled in barley water, until they become of a redish colour, then take them out and beat them with shells in a mortar, till they are as soft as mash, let the juice be poured out, and given to the patient in an equal quantity of chicken broth, or any other broth that is not too strong.

THE COMPLEAT VERMIN KILLER AND USEFUL POCKET COMPANION, DUBLIN 1778.

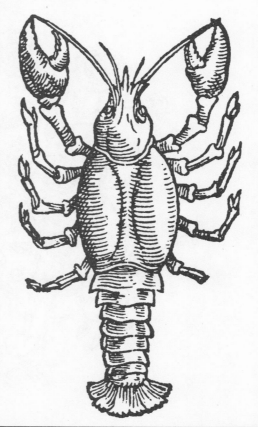

A GOOD WATER FOR CONSUMPTION: Take a peck of green garden snails, wash them in bear (beer) put them in an oven and let stand till they've done crying; then with a knife and fork prick the green from them, and beat the snailshells and all in a stone mortar. Then take a quart of green earth-worms, slice them thru the middle and strow them with salt; then wash them and beat them, the pot being first put into the still with two handfuls of angelico, a quart of rosemary flowers, then the snails and worms, the egrimony, bearsfeet, red dock roots, barbery brake, bilbony, wormwood, of each two handfuls. One handful of red tumerick and one ounce of saffron, well dried and beaten. Then pour in three gallons of milk. Wait till morning, then put in three cloves, (well beaten) hartshorn, grated. Keep the still covered all night. This done, stir it not. Distil with a moderate fire. The patient must take two spoonfuls at a time.

AN HISTORICAL ALMANAC OF CANADA

The preceding recipe comes from a 17th century cookbook of Mrs. Edward Wolfe, mother of Brigadier-General James Wolfe, victorious commander of the British troops against the French in Quebec in 1759.

Reverend Wesley, as usual, will have the last word.

TAKE A COW HEEL from the tripe house, ready dressed, two quarts of new milk, two ounces of hartshorn shavings, two ounces of isinglass, a quarter of a pound of sugar candy and a race of ginger. Put all these into a pot and set it in the oven after the bread is drawn. Let it continue there till the oven is nearly cold; and let the patient live on this. I have known this cure a deep consumptive more than once.

OR, every morning cut up a little turf of fresh earth and lying down, breath into the hole for a quarter of an hour. I have known a deep consumptive cured thus. In the last stage, suck a healthy woman daily. This cured my father.

REVEREND JOHN WESLEY, *PRIMITIVE PHYSICK*, 1747

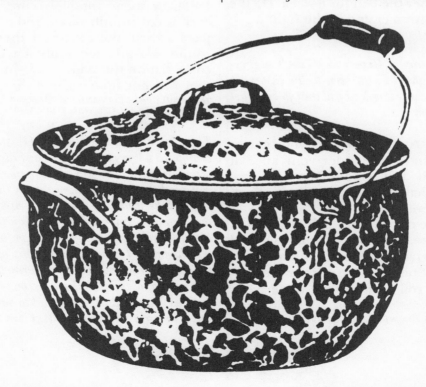

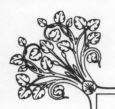

Cramps

I'll rock thee with old cramps,
Fill all thy bones with aches.
SHAKESPEARE, *THE TEMPEST*

These folk cures for cramps are quite similar, except you would be in real trouble with the Texas remedy if you owned only one pair of shoes . . . either cramps or bare feet for a week.

TO CURE CRAMPS IN THE FEET, turn your shoes upside down before going to bed.
APPALACHIAN FOLK REMEDY

TO CURE CRAMPS IN THE LEGS, take the last pair of shoes you had on and if the cramp is in the left leg, take the left shoe and put it in the right shoe and place them under the bed for a week. Do the opposite for a cramp in the right leg.
TEXAS REMEDY

If you try any of Reverend Wesley's suggestions, you should also turn to the insomnia section, because it is doubtful that you will get much sleep.

CRAMPS, TO PREVENT: Tie your garter smooth and tight under your knee at going to bed. It seldom fails.
OR, take half a pint of tar-water morning and evening.
OR, to one ounce and a half of spirits of turpentine, add flour of brimstone and sulphur vivum, of each half an ounce: smell it at night, three or four times.
OR, lay a roll of brimstone under your pillow.
REVEREND JOHN WESLEY, *PRIMITIVE PHYSICK,* 1747

Here are two cures which involve wearing certain paraphernalia to ward off the cramp.

AN AMULET AGAINST CRAMP: Take white root of rhubarb, pulverize the same, and fill with such powder a square pouch made of linen, about three thumbs in size. The patient should carry the pouch on a string around his neck that it will touch the bare skin in the neighbourhood of the stomach.
ALBERTUS MAGNUS OR EGYPTIAN SECRETS

IN ITALY, as an infallible cure, a new cork is cut in thin slices, and a riband passed thru' the centre of them, tied round the affected limb. Laying the corks flat on the skin; while thus worn they prevent any return of the cramp.
THE FAMILY PHYSICIAN AND THE FARMER'S COMPANION, SYRACUSE, NEW YORK, 1840

The Family Magazine, *1741, described cramps as a 'very troublesome disorder that is often attended with bad consequences.' After you read the recipe, you might say that having to take medicine with oil of earthworms was bad consequences! To save you the trouble of searching for a good recipe for Oil of Earthworms, I am including this one: Put the earthworms into a pot and wrap the same up in a loaf of bread, bake it in a bake oven as long as it is necessary for bread to bake, then put it in a glass vessel and distil it in the sun.*

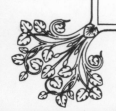
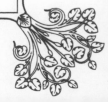

RECEIPT FOR THE CRAMP: Take ointment of marshmallows, oil of worms, of each half an ounce; oil of turpentine, two drachms; camphire, two scruples; compound spirit of lavender, two drachms; oil of cloves, six drops: make a linement and anoint the part affected well with a warm hand.
THE FAMILY MAGAZINE, LONDON 1741

Tonight thou shalt have cramps,
Side-stitches that shall pen thy breathe up.
SHAKESPEARE, *THE TEMPEST*

A STITCH IN THE SIDE: Apply apple treacle spread on hot toast (tried).
REVEREND JOHN WESLEY, *PRIMITIVE PHYSICK,* 1747

A stiff neck is a special type of cramp with its own special cures.

CRICK IN THE NECK: Go down to the hog pen and watch until a hog has rubbed its neck against the fence, then rub your neck in the same spot and the crick will disappear.
TEXAS REMEDY

TO CURE CRISS IN THE NECK: As soon as you find your neck stiff or turned to one side by the contraction of nerves, apply over the place diseased a piece of black oil-cloth, with the right side to the skin, and then with a thick handkerchief tie up the neck; in a short time the part will grow moist, and by leaving it thus during the night or through the day, the pain will be removed.
U.S. PRACTICAL RECEIPT BOOK, 1844.

WEAR A POT HOOK around the neck to cure a crick in the neck. To avert cramp in the legs, place a pair of scissors or some other piece of steel in your bed.
KENTUCKY FOLK REMEDY

And be careful not to roll over!

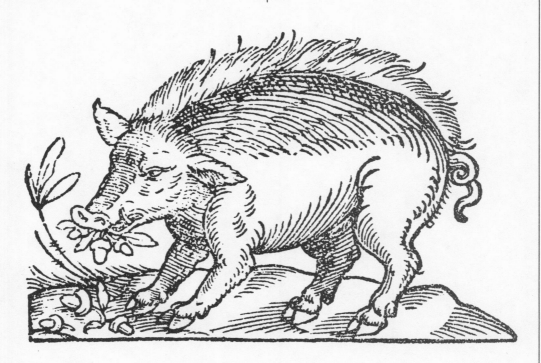

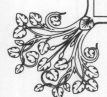

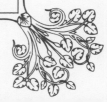

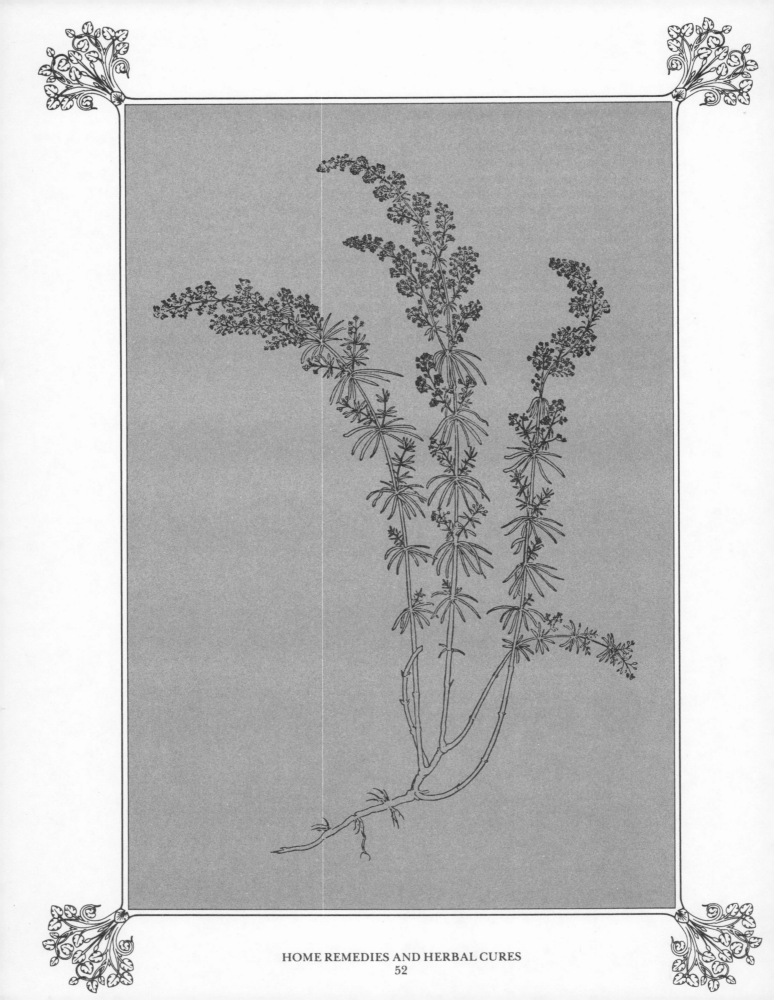

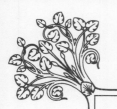

Croup

Eat no green apples or you'll droop,
Be careful not to get the croup,
Avoid the chicken-pox and such,
And don't fall out of windows much.
EDWARD ANTHONY, *ADVICE TO SMALL CHILDREN*

Croup is a household term given to a group of diseases characterized by swelling or partial blockage of the entrance of the larynx. It attacks children. Most of the following remedies work on the theory that the child should be made to vomit to open the passage.

TAKE THE WHITE OF HEN DUNG, steep it in soft water, not boil it, strain and dissolve in loaf sugar. Dose one teaspoonful often as the case requires. It will evacuate the stomach and bowels. Tried.
A NUMBER OF RECEIPTS FOR CURING MAN AND BEAST, 1855

FOR A SUDDEN ATTACK OF QUINCY OR CROUP, bathe the neck with bear's grease and pour it down the throat. A linen rag soaked in sweet oil, butter or lard and sprinkled with yellow scotch snuff is said to have performed wonderful cures in cases of croup. It should be placed where the distress is greatest.
CANADIAN PIONEER RECIPE

A PIECE OF FRESH LARD, as large as a butternut, rubbed up with sugar, in the same way that butter and sugar are prepared for the dressing of puddings, divided into three parts, and given at intervals of twenty minutes, will relieve any case of croup not already allowed to progress to the fatal point.
AVERY'S ALMANACK, SAINT JOHN, NEW BRUNSWICK, 1857

Dr Chase appears to have sensed some scepticism over his cures and admonished his readers. 'Many people will stick up their noses at these "Old Grandmother prescriptions" but I tell many "Upstart" physicians that our grandmothers are carrying more information out of the world by their deaths than will ever be possessed by this class of "sniffers", and I really thank God, so do thousands of others, that He has enabled me, in this work to redeem such an amount of it for the benefit of the world.'

DUTCH REMEDY: Goose oil and urine, equal quantities. Dose: from one teaspoon to a tablespoon of the mixture according to the age of the child. Repeat the dose every fifteen minutes if the first dose doesn't vomit in that time.
DR CHASE'S RECIPES, 1867 EDITION

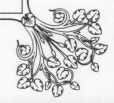
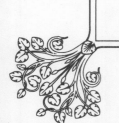

Most of these croup cures would make children agree with Francis Bacon's comment that 'the remedy is worse than the disease.' In the case of this remedy using calomel, the cure could be deadly or debilitating for life.

A DOSE OF CALOMEL will almost always break up croup. Have it issued in doses, according to age, by your druggist.
INGLENOOK DOCTOR BOOK, 1911

Calomel is a sad story in the history of medicine. It is a mercury compound which was used from the 16th century until after the end of the American Civil War, when it was recognized to be a deadly poison. It was an emetic (vomit-producing) and used for a wide variety of complaints. In giving massive doses of the compound, doctors were ignorantly inflicting acute mercury poisoning on their patients. If they recovered from the original ailment, they spent the rest of their lives suffering from the deterioration of their nervous system.

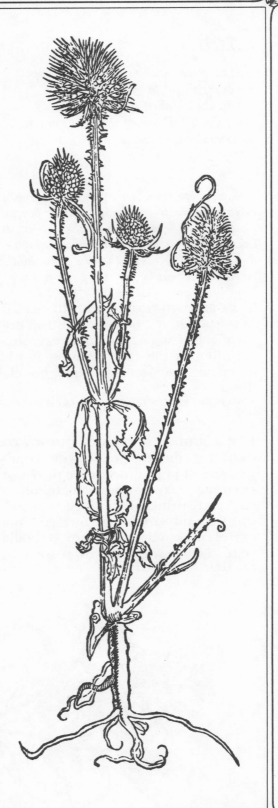

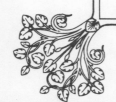

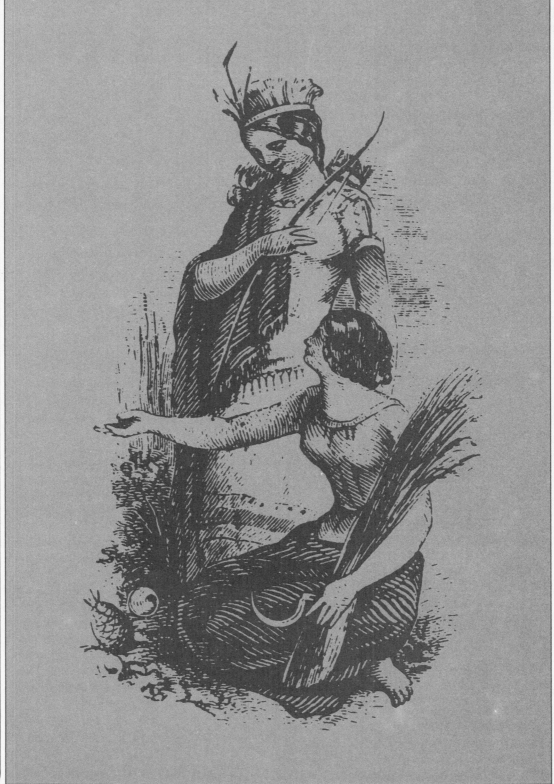

Deafness

Deaf, giddy, helpless, left alone,
To all my friends a burden grown,
No more I hear my church's bell
Than if it rang out for my knell;
At thunder now no more I start
Than at the rumbling of a cart,
And what's incredible, alack!
No more I hear a woman's clack.

JONATHAN SWIFT (1667-1745) ON HIS OWN DEAFNESS

If Jonathan Swift had known Albertus Magnus's remedy and climbed to the top of St. Patrick's Cathedral in Dublin, where he was Dean, he might never have had to write a poem on deafness.

FOR BAD HEARING: Take the oil with which the bells of churches are greased, and smear it behind the afflicted ears, and relief will not fail to come at once.
ALBERTUS MAGNUS OR EGYPTIAN SECRETS

The next ingredients are nothing if not natural products. Urine has long been a popular cure for chilblains, earaches, corns and warts.

TO CURE DEAFNESS AND NOISE IN THE HEAD: Put your own urine into a pewter dish and cover it with another, then put some coals under and when it is hot, brush off the clear water that hangs on the upper dish with a feather and drop into the ear; this hath done great cures.
OR
Ram's urine, eel's bile and juice of ash expressed and placed in the ears.
OLD ENGLISH REMEDY

TAKE ANT'S EGGS and onion juice; mix; and drop into the ear: or, drop into the ear, at night, six or eight drops of warm chamber lye.
LADIES INDISPENSABLE ASSISTANT, NEW YORK, 1851

The Ladies Indispensable Assistant *was being 'delicate' when it described urine as chamber lye.*

AN APPROVED REMEDY FOR A PRESENT DEAFNESS: Take of the breast milk of a woman that has had her first male-child some time before, and drop three or four drops of it warm, as it comes from the nipple, into the part affected.
THE COMPLETE FAMILY PIECE AND COUNTRY GENTLEMAN AND FARMER'S BEST GUIDE, LONDON, 1741

(The Texans recommended washing sore eyes in breast milk, and Reverend Wesley swore that his father was saved from the last stages of consumption by suckling a healthy woman.)

While human urine and breast milk are readily accessible and cost nothing, the ingredients in the next two may be more difficult to locate. In the 16th century, Shakespeare could write 'Give me an ounce of civet, good apothecary, to sweeten my imagination'; your druggist today would be hard-pressed to supply civet—the musky-smelling ingredient found in the anal glands of a weasel-like animal. It was once widely used in perfumes.

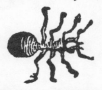

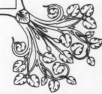

TO CURE DEAFNESS: Take clean, fine black wool, dip it in civet and put it into the ear, as it dries, which in a day or two it will, dip into again and keep it moistened in the ear for three weeks or a month.

U.S. PRACTICAL RECEIPT BOOK, 1844

AN ANCIENT CURE: Have the fat from the kidneys of wild rabbit, gridel it out and put in two drops in each ear, each night, rub cotton batting to a point, dip it in the immediate relief and put it in the ear. Let it remain till better.

MRS PALMER'S HOME REMEDY BOOK, QUOTED IN AN HISTORICAL ALMANAC OF CANADA

The following was brought to Newfoundland in 1841 with Mrs Benjamin Smith and her medical missionary husband. Mrs Smith had inherited the family doctor book at the time of her wedding. The original notebook is in the Newfoundland provincial archives.

FOR DEAFNESS WHEN OCCASIONED BY THE WAX HARDENING IN THE EARS: Take the inside of a cabbage stalk, that part which runs up the middle of the leaf, cut the outside off and put a little of the inside into the ear at night. Then take it out and with a syringe inject a little milk and warm water after which put a little cotton wool into the ear to prevent taking cold.

MRS (REVEREND) B. SMITH, NEWFOUNDLAND

Or, try these in your ear:

PUT GROUND IVY one leafe into each ear rowle it up but not too hard put it in fresh morning and evenings.

A BOOK OF SIMPLES, LONDON, c. 1750

Ground ivy is also known as Gill-go-over-the-ground, alehoof or haymaids.

TO CURE DEAFNESS: Take a clove of garlick, and roast it very soft: then take a few drops of oil of bitter almonds and mix with it and a little saffron; mix this all together in a spoon and put it into a bag, and put the bag into the ear, fresh and as warm as can be suffered. Take this out in the morning and stop the ear with black wool from a sheep and be careful of taking cold; and continue this for a fortnight. This is a pattern of the bag, both as to shape and size, with a string to it.

THE FAMILY MAGAZINE, LONDON, 1741

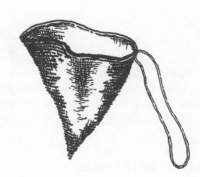

DEAFNESS: If Recent to Cure, if not, to Relieve: Hen's oil, one gill; and a single handful of the sweet clover raised in gardens; stew it in the oil until the juice is all out, strain it and bottle for use. When deafness is recent, it will be cured by putting three or four drops daily into the ear, but if of long standing, much relief will be obtained if continued a sufficient length of time.

DR CHASE'S RECIPES, 1867 EDITION

I wish Dr Chase would have explained how he proposed to 'relieve' deafness without curing it.

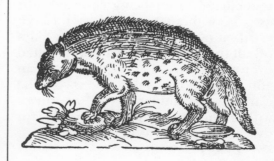

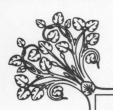

Diarrhea and Dysentery

Of all the home remedies, a good wife is the best.
KIN HUBBARD (1868-1930)

Buckeye Cookery, *a little cookbook from Minneapolis, gave the following advice to wives. 'Bad dinners go hand in hand with total depravity, while a properly fed man is already half saved.' Careless wives were told that*

CHRONIC DIARRHEA: Is cured by drinking orange peel tea, sweetened with loaf-sugar, and use as a common drink for twenty-four or thirty-six hours.
BUCKEYE COOKERY, 1881

INDIAN REMEDY: Make a decoction of spruce tops, sweetened with loaf sugar; take half a teacupful once an hour. Sometimes, the medicine taken for this disorder produces pain, and constipation of the bowels, owing to the sudden check which is produced, a dose of rhubarb is required.
THE PEOPLE'S MANUAL, WORCESTER, MASSACHUSETTS, 1848

TAKE SOME BUTTER off the churn, immediately after being churned, just as it is, without be salted or washed; clarify it over the fire like honey. Skim off all the milky particles when melted over a clear fire. Let the patient (if an adult) take two tablespoons of the clarified remainder, twice or thrice within the day...A simple cure for dysentery which has never failed.
THE CANADA FARMER, TORONTO, 28 AUGUST 1847

DIARRHEA: Laudanum, a quarter ounce, wintergreen, half an ounce, oil of anise, half an ounce, Brandy eight ounces. Dose: One teaspoon every hour till checked. For children, two years: dose: One-quarter teaspoon.
CANADIAN PIONEER REMEDY

CHEAPER AND BETTER CURE: Aromatic syrup of rhubarb. Dose: Tablespoon every hour until checked.
CANADIAN PIONEER REMEDY

Laudanum is a liquid opium solution. Another opium and anise mixture, paregoric, is still considered by many doctors today to be a very effective cure for diarrhea. Paregoric, however, can only be obtained by prescription.

POMEGRANATE BARK: This bark is a valuable remedy to have on hand in the far bush where doctors and nurses are distant and dysentery or diarrhea are common complaints. The ordinary mixture is made by boiling half an ounce of dried bark of pomegranate fruit in half a pint of water; one tablespoonful of the infusion to be given every three hours.
THE KOOKABURRA COOKERY BOOK.

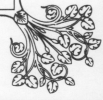

This newspaper clipping was in a scrapbook of medical recipes collected by a Canadian pioneer.

PARCH A HALF PINT of rice until it is perfectly brown. Boil it down as it is usually done, and eat it slowly, and it will check, if not entirely stop, the most violent diarrhea in a few hours. Ordinarily, a little brandy, say half a wineglassful, with loaf sugar dissolved in it will have the same effect. However, it is better in all cases to avoid alcohol as a medicine if other antidotes can be had. In the more obstinate cases, where brandy is used, its efficacy is increased by stirring it with a red hot iron.

Dysentery, also known in the past as bloody flux, is, mercifully, less common today in many parts of the world. The lack of sanitation, refrigeration for food or knowledge about germs, made it a universal complaint in past ages. Neither strewing herbs on the ground to ward off disease nor the following cures would have done much to relieve the victims.

TAKE PIG'S DUNG, dry it and burn it to grey (not white) Ashes; of these give about half a dram for a dose, drinking after them about three spoonfuls of Wine Vinegar.
THE COMPLETE FAMILY PIECE AND COUNTRY GENTLEMAN AND FARMER'S BEST GUIDE, LONDON, 1741

FOR THE DYSENTERY AND PLEURISY: Grate to a fine powder the dry'd Pizzle of a Stag, and give of it as much as will be upon a Shilling or thereabouts, once or twice a day in any convenient Vehicle.
THE COMPLETE FAMILY PIECE AND COUNTRY GENTLEMAN AND FARMER'S BEST GUIDE, LONDON, 1741

Pizzle means the penis of the stag. I really don't know where one goes for powdered Stag pizzle these days.

FOR DYSENTERY AND DIARRHEA: Take the moss off of trees and boil it in red wine and let those that are affected with these diseases, drink it.
THE LONG LOST FRIEND, 1856

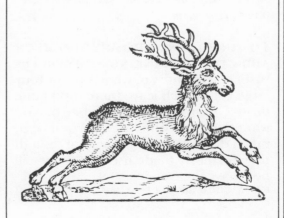

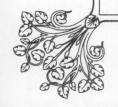
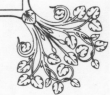

Drunkenness

Not drunk is he who from the floor
Can rise alone, and still drink more;
But drunk is he who prostrate lies,
Without the power to drink or rise.

T.L. PEACOCK, *MISFORTUNES OF ELPHIN*

Not everyone would agree with Peacock's definition of drunkenness. Temperance groups, for example, tended to expound the belief that even taking a sip of liquor was a huge step down the road to ruin. To quote a verse from the English parody and occasional rugby tune called 'The Song of the Temperance Union'.

> We do not eat fruitcake because it has rum
> And one little bite turns a man to a bum.
> Can you imagine a sorrier sight
> Than a man eating fruitcake
> Until he gets tight.

Considering that this position was probably held by most people at a temperance meeting on 22 February 1842, it must have taken some courage for Abraham Lincoln to pronounce, 'If we take habitual drunkards as a class, their heads and their hearts will bear an advantageous comparison with those of any other class.' But however kind and intelligent drunks may be, there is still an obsession to cure them.

TO CURE THOSE WHO ARE TOO MUCH ADDICTED TO DRINKING WINE: Put in a sufficient quantity of wine three or four large eels, which leave there until quite dead. Give that wine to the person you want to reform and he or she will be so much disgusted with wine, that though they formerly made use of it, they will now have an aversion to it.
U.S. PRACTICAL RECEIPT BOOK, 1844

TO WEAN A TIPPLER FROM DRINKING WINE: Take an apple, put it into the hand of a dying man, and let the apple remain there till the person dies. If you desire the tippler to drink only half the quantity he usually takes, give him one half of the apple to eat; but if you wish him to abstain totally from strong drinks give him the entire apple to eat. But the drunkard must not be aware of your designs.
ALBERTUS MAGNUS OR EGYPTIAN SECRETS

TO KEEP A FEEBLE BRAIN FROM DRUNKENNESS: Take in the morning fasting five leaves of betony and eat them and keep some in your hand to smell there (at) all the day and you will be saved.
STERE ITT WELL

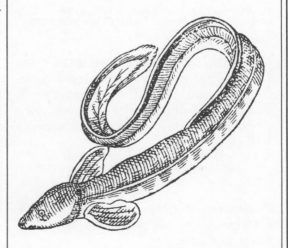

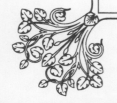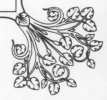

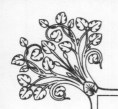

The best cure for drunkenness is, sober, to look at a drunken man.
CHINESE PROVERB

The following tonics and teas show more sympathy for the addict than does the shock tactic of eels in the wineglass.

NEW GERMAN REMEDY FOR TIPPLING: Take one teaspoonful of the tincture of calumba, one teaspoonful of the tincture of cascarilla, one teaspoonful of the compound of gentian, a wine-glassful of infusion of quassia, twenty drops of elixor of vitriol. Mix and take twice or thrice a day, and have a jug of cold water dashed over the head every morning on coming out of bed, and the feet bathed in warm water every night. Continue this for six or eight weeks.
THE FAMILY ORACLE OF HEALTH, ECONOMY, MEDICINE AND GOOD LIVING, LONDON, 1825

Elixir of vitriol was invented in the 17th century by a German doctor, Adrian Mynsicht, and was a pungent mixture composed of cinnamon, ginger, cloves, nutmeg, sage, mint, cubels, aloes, lemon peel, calamus, aromaticus, galengal root and sugar.

TO CURE A PERSON'S THIRST FOR ARDENT SPIRITS: Take blood root, pods of Indian tobacco dried and pulverized, of each a teaspoonful, which should be put into a pint of the spirit you like best: and whenever you thirst for liquor, drink a swallow of this and you will soon be cured of that pernicious habit.
THE FAMILY PHYSICIAN AND FARMER'S COMPANION, SYRACUSE, NEW YORK, 1840

THERE IS A PRESCRIPTION in use in England for the cure of drunkenness, by which thousands are said to have been assisted in recovering themselves. It is as follows: sulphate of iron, five grains; peppermint water, eleven drachms; spirit of nutmeg, one drachm: twice a day. This preparation acts as a stimulant and tonic and partially supplies the place of the accustomed liquor and prevents the absolute physical and moral prostration that follows a sudden cessation from the use of stimulating drinks.
BUCKEYE COOKERY, MINNEAPOLIS, 1881

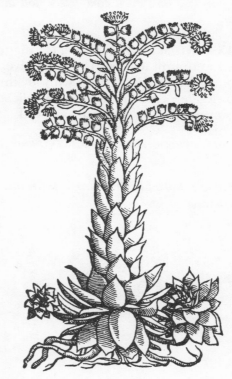

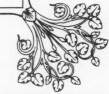

THOMPSON'S COMPOSITION TEA: It is claimed that Thompson's composition tea will cure drunkenness. Take hemlock bark, one pound; bay berry bark, two pounds; ginger root, one pound; cloves, two ounces; and cayenne pepper, two ounces: pulverize and mix well. Of this take half a teaspoonful with a teaspoonful of sugar and put into half a teacupful of boiling water. After it has stood a few minutes fill the cup with milk. Drink half of this upon rising in the morning and the rest just before meal time.
THE PEOPLE'S HOME MEDICAL BOOK, CLEVELAND, OHIO, 1916

Even these remedies would probably make castor oil taste good. And maybe it was the threat of having such foul potions forced down their throats that convinced some drunks to abstain. But if the other recipes failed, there was always this surefire remedy which would either cure the addict or kill him—since stramonium contains an alkaloid called daturine which in large doses can paralyze and even completely stop the heart.

STRAMONIUM LEAVES: Give a tea made of stramonium leaves. It may be given in tea or coffee, if desired without the knowledge of the patient. Will relieve the appetite for tobacco as well as liquor.
THE PEOPLE'S HOME MEDICAL BOOK, CLEVELAND, OHIO, 1916

There are more old drunkards than old physicians.

RABELAIS, 1535

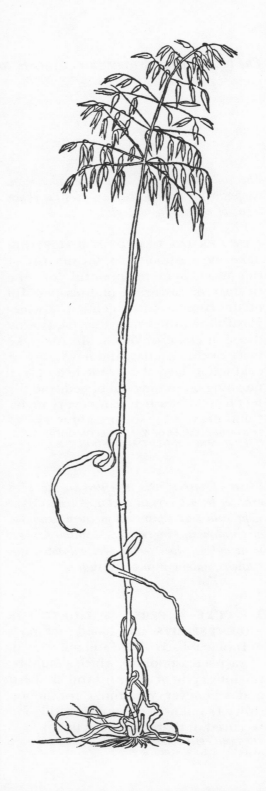

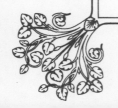

Earaches
(Also see deafness)

Nature has given man one tongue, but two ears, that we may hear twice as much as we speak.
EPICTETUS

We often don't acknowledge this logic, nor do we thank Nature very much when both our ears are aching. In the 18th century, that cure-all, opium, was a popular prescription for earaches.

EAR-ACHE AND DEAFNESS, VALUABLE REMEDY: Wine of opium (not laudanum), one dram; oil of anise, ten drops: put into an ounce bottle and fill with oil of sweet almonds (sweet oil will do as well). Directions: shake well and drop from three to five drops into the ear, or ears; if both are affected. If no relief in five to ten minutes, repeat, and follow along to relieve the sound of roaring in the ears.
DR CHASE'S RECIPES, 1892 EDITION

COTTON WET WITH SWEET OIL and paregoric relieves the earache very soon. The negroes, at the south, consider a cockroach cut in two and applied to the ear, the most certain cure for the earache.
THE LADY'S ANNUAL REGISTER, BOSTON 1838

The next remedy does not say where you put the cotton—over the ears? or over the nose?

MIXTURE OF EQUAL PARTS of chloroform and laudanum, a little being introduced on a piece of cotton. The first effect is a sensation of cold, then numbness, followed by scarcely perceptible pain and refreshing sleep.
THE CANADA FARMER, TORONTO, 15 JUNE 1864

Quite often earaches are caused by a build-up of wax. St. Jean de la Salle (1651-1719) in his book The Rules of Christian Manners and Civility *gave this misguided advice on how to keep the ears clean: 'The ears should be kept perfectly clean; but it must never be done in company. It should never be done with a pin, and still less with the fingers, but always with an ear-picker.' Nothing is more dangerous than sticking a sharp object in the ear. However, some of the next cures using warm oil are far more sensible suggestions for dislodging hard wax.*

FOR A PAIN IN THE EAR: Take the juice of mountain sage, oil of fennel, or oil of olives, and mix well together; drop into the pained ear three drops for several nights. It will ease and draw out any imposthume if that be the cause.
U.S. PRACTICAL RECEIPT BOOK, 1844

INDIAN CURE: Take a piece of lean mutton, the size of a large walnut, put it into the fire and burn it for some time till it is reduced almost to a cinder; then put it into a piece of clean rag, and squeeze it until some moisture is expressed which must be dropped into the ear as hot as a patient can stand it.
DR CHASE'S RECIPES, 1880 EDITION

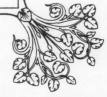

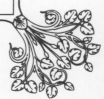

PEACH SEEDS, GLYCERINE AND SWEET OIL: Take the kernels from nine peach seeds, pound them up fine, put into a small vessel and add one tablespoonful of glycerine or sweet oil and cook until the kernels are of a dark brown colour; then strain and it is ready for use. The dose is one or two drops in the ear. Repeat every hour, if necessary, until relieved. The person sending this recipe adds: 'This is a sure and tried remedy as we have used it in our family for sixteen years and have never had to use it over three times in any case. When you haven't the sweet oil or glycerine as called for, you can use castor oil.'
THE PEOPLE'S HOME MEDICAL BOOK, CLEVELAND, OHIO, 1916

Two and a half centuries earlier, herbalist Nicholas Culpeper had also advocated using the oil from kernels of peach stones to stop earaches. He further recommended that 'if the kernels be bruised and applied to the head, it marvellously procures the hair to grow again upon·bald places, or where it is thin.'

The Texans suggest pecan oil. However, they offer some less pleasant alternatives.

TEXAS REMEDIES
• Urinate on your finger and stick the finger in your ear.
• Fill ear with mud made from bird droppings.
• Heat salt and place in the end of a sock. Put the sock on the ear.
• Hold a baby over a hogpen to cure its earache.

Some remedies suggested immersing the feet in warm water as part of an earache cure. Perhaps the treat of warm feet offsets the pain of the earache?

SOAK THE FEET in warm water; roast an onion and put the heart of it into the ear as warm as it can be borne; heat a brick and wrap it up and apply to the side of the head. When the feet are taken from the water, bind roasted onions on them. Lard or sweet oil, dropped into the ear, as warm as it can be borne, is good.
BROCKVILLE ALMANAC, 1866

PUT INTO THE EAR a clove of garlic or a small fig toasted and bathe the feet in warm water at bedtime, taking care to stop the ears with undressed wool and to keep the head very warm at night.
THE HOUSEKEEPER'S ALMANAC, NEW YORK, 1842

These advertised instant and immediate relief:

TAKE A BIT of cotton batting, put upon it a pinch of black pepper, gather it up and tie it, dip in sweet oil and insert it in the ear. Put a flannel bandage over the head to keep it warm. It will give immediate relief.
THE FARMER'S ADVOCATE, LONDON, ONTARIO, AUGUST 1876

TAKE A LARGE ONION and cut it into slices; put a slice of onion; then a slice (the author would say a piece of leaf the size of the onion) of strong tobacco, then a slice of onion again, then tobacco, until the onion is all laid up, then wrap in a wet cloth and cover in hot embers until the onion is cooked; press out the juice with heavy pressure and drop into the ear. It give instant relief.
DR CHASE'S RECIPES, 1892 EDITION

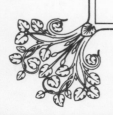

In London, The Family Magazine *warned of the alarming consequences of earwigs, for it was common belief that these nasty insects could burrow through the ear into the head. This belief is not true although earwigs do exist and do like to live in ears.*

EASY METHOD FOR ATTRACTING EARWIGS FROM THE EAR: A person lately having an earwig crept into his ear, and knowing the particular fondness that insect has for apples, immediately applied a piece of apple to the ear, which enticed the creature out, and thereby prevented the alarming consequences which might have otherwise ensued.

OR

FOR AN EAR-WIG HAVING GOTTEN INTO THE EAR: Take rue and stamp it in a mortar, then strain off the juice and put it into the ear; then lie down to rest on the contrary ear, and when you awake, the juice will come out, and the ear-wig will be dead.

The juice of wormwood, of southernwood, and rue, of equal quantity, put into the ear, will also kill any vermin that has got into it.

THE FAMILY MAGAZINE, LONDON, 1741

TO KILL EARWIGS OR OTHER INSECTS, WHICH MAY ACCIDENTLY HAVE CREPT INTO THE EAR: Let the person under this distressing circumstance lay his head upon a table the side upwards that is afflicted: at the same time let some friend carefully drop into the ear a little sweet oil, or oil of almonds. A drop or two will be sufficient which will instantly destroy the insect and remove the pain, however violent.

NEW FAMILY RECEIPT BOOK, LONDON, 1815

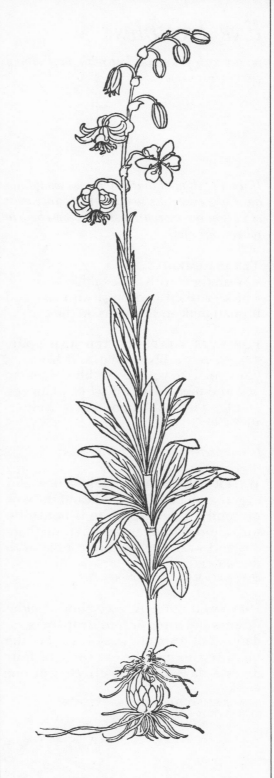

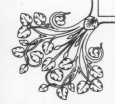

Eye Troubles

Never rub your eyes but with your elbow
ENGLISH PROVERB

If we all followed that advice, we would not have sore eyes quite so often. But, since most of us ignore wise counsel, here is some help to relieve our eyes.

TEXAS REMEDIES:
• Wash them with breast milk.
• Mix crushed bed bugs with salt and human milk and rub this on the eyes.

FOR EYES THAT ARE RED AND SORE: Take a red cabbage leaf and bruise it (and put it) to your eyes when you go to bed and mix it with the white of an egg and let it lie so all night and it heals.
STERE ITT WELL

If you prefer your eggs hard-boiled,

WATER FOR THE EYES: Take a new laid egg, roast it blue-hard, take out the yolk presently while the white is hot, fill it with alum and sugar candy; strain them out and wash the eye twice a day with the water.
THE FAMILY MAGAZINE, LONDON, 1741

INFLAMED EYES: A decoction of elder flowers and three or four drops of laundanum, to a small glass of tea. Let the mixture run into the eye three or four times a day. A cure is effected in one week.
FARMER'S DIRECTORY AND HOUSEKEEPER'S ASSISTANT, TORONTO, 1851

EYE SALVES: Wine and pepper. Put a horn-cup and into the eyes when thou wilt and go to rest. Take strawberry plant, the lower part, and pepper. Put into a cloth; tie up; steep in sweetened wine. Drip one drop from the cloth into either eye. This is the best eyesalve. Take bumble-bees honey, and foxes grease, and roe-bucks marrow. Mix together.
LACNUNGA, 10TH C. EARLY ANGLO-SAXON REMEDIES

A REMEDY FOR INFLAMMED EYES: Mix one dram of salt of tartar with a pint of frog's spawn; let them dissolve together and annoint the eyes with the composition several times every day till the inflammation is removed.
THE COMPLEAT VERMIN KILLER AND USEFUL POCKET COMPANION, DUBLIN, 1778

In Milton's Paradise Lost, *the Archangel Michael, after Adam's Fall, anointed his eyes with a mixture of eyebright and rue along with Three Drops from the Well of Life. Even with the Archangel Michael's, or at least Milton's, endorsement, there has been dispute over the effectiveness of the eyebright plant. Herbalist Nicholas Culpeper sided with the great prince of all angels. As he wrote in* The English Physician: *If the herb was but as much used at it is neglected, it would spoil the spectacle maker's trade.' The next four remedies believe in the power of eyebright.*

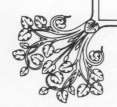
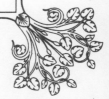

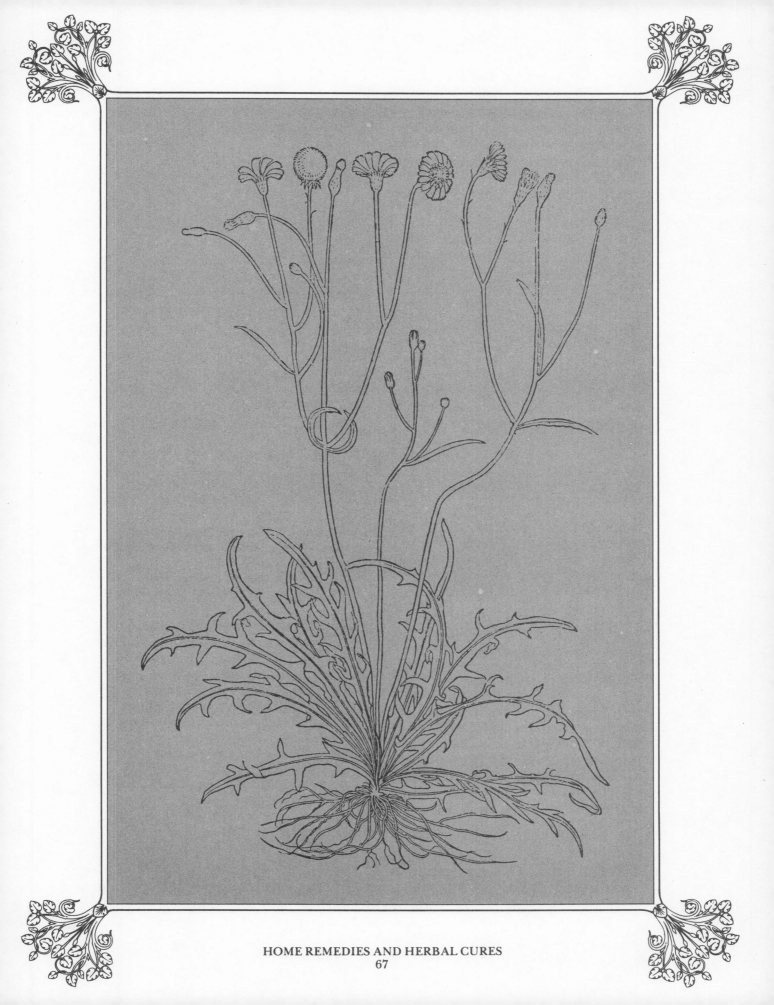

THE LADY FITZHARDING'S EYE WATER WHICH LATELY CUR'D AN ALMOST BLIND PERSON WHOSE EYES LOOK'D LIKE GLASS: Take three spoonfuls of white rose water, as much eye-bright water, and as much sifted white sugar candy as will lie on a three pence and the same quantity of fine aloes, sifted and put to the water, and shak'd together, and drop a few drops every night going to bed.
THE FAMILY MAGAZINE, LONDON, 1741

TO RECOVER OR STRENGTHEN A WEAK EYE SIGHT: Take of cloves, nutmeg grains of each half an ounce, of English saffron, two pennyworth, of eye-bright leaves dryed in the sun, a handfull, make all these into fine powder, then take eight or nine raisons of ye sun, stone them, then put into every of them as much of the powder as will lye on a penny, eating them in a morning fasting not eating an hour after.
A BOOK OF SIMPLES, LONDON, *c*. 1750

INFLAMMATION OF THE EYES: Mix bread crumbs with the white of an egg, three drops of brandy and a very little salt. Apply in a bag of thin soft linen or muslin. It is better to apply it at night when lying down. It always affords relief. Drink also eye-bright tea and wash eyes with it.
DR CHASE'S RECIPES, 1880 EDITION

DR MORIATY'S EYE-WATER: Take white rose water, plantain water, and eye-bright, of each one ounce and an half, verjuice, half an ounce, prepar'd tutty, half a drachm: mix all these together with the white of an egg.
THE FAMILY MAGAZINE, LONDON, 1741

Tutty is a crude zinc oxide once used in medicines and now used as a polishing powder.

*And all eyes
Blind with pin and web but theirs
   —theirs only,
That would unseen be wicked.*
SHAKESPEARE, *THE WINTER'S TALE*

Pin and web was the Elizabethan expression to describe what was quite likely a cataract. And no matter how exotic the ingredients, cataracts and films over the eye could not be cured. Only today with exquisitely delicate surgery can cataracts be removed. But still, people tried to restore the victim's sight with the following.

TO REMOVE FILMS FROM THE EYES: Take of powder of pearls and powder of coral, each an ounce, one dram of crab's eyes, two ounces of virgin honey, and let them all be mixed together as an ointment, which must be applied to the eyes morning and evening, and often if necessary.
THE COMPLEAT VERMIN KILLER AND USEFUL POCKET COMPANION, DUBLIN, 1778

CATARACT ON THE EYE: Apply the oil of a rabbit twice a day for a week or two. The same is good for sore eyes.
A NUMBER OF RECEIPTS FOR CURING MAN AND BEAST, 1855

THE JUICE OF CELANDINE, field daisies and ground ivy, clariefied and a little fine sugar dissolved therein and dropped into the eyes, is a sovereign remedy for all pains, redness and watering of them; as also for pin and web, skins and films growing over the sight; it helpth beast as well as men.
NICHOLAS CULPEPER, THE ENGLISH PHYSICIAN, 1652

Culpeper explained that celandine comes from the Greek word meaning swallow, because they say if you put out the eyes of young swallows when they are in the nest, the older birds will pluck celandine to restore their offsprings' sight.

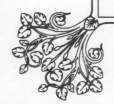
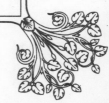

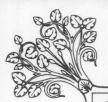

GOOD FOR EYES: To give brilliancy to the eyes, shut them early at night, and open them early in the morning; let the mind be constantly intent on acquisition of benevolent feelings. This will scarcely ever fail to impart to the eyes an intelligent and amiable expression.
DR CHASE'S RECIPES, 1880 EDITION

But, knowing his readers and their frailties, he provided other recipes as well.

APPLY AS A POULTICE boiled, roasted or rotten apples, warm. Or wormwood tops with a yolk of an egg. This will hardly fail. Or, beat the white of an egg with two spoonfuls of white rose water into a white froth. Apply this on a fine rag, changing it so that it may not grow dry till the eye or eyelid is well. Tried.
DR CHASE'S RECIPES, 1880 EDITION

I suspect Dr Chase pinched the above from Reverend Wesley's book without giving him due credit. However, he volunteered that the next one was given to him, highly recommended, by an old Scottish sailor who used it when nothing else was available.

SAILOR'S EYE PREPARATION: Burn alum and mix with it the whites of eggs, and put between two clothes and lay it upon the eyes; taking salts and cream of tartar equal parts, to cleanse the blood.
DR CHASE'S RECIPES, 1867 EDITION

Cicero said, 'The keenest of all our senses is the sense of sight,' and to improve that sense, a 17th century remedy suggests,

TO STRENGTHEN YE EYES: Let another that is young chow annyseeds and then breathe upon ye party's eyes.
THE RECEIPT BOOK OF MRS ANN BLENCOWE, 1694

Lying is bad for your health in more ways than one. It was believed to be the cause of hiccoughs and, according to Texan folklore, the cause of sties in the eye. Of course, the Texans have lots of suggestions on how to cure this painful inflammation of the eyelid.

TEXAS REMEDIES
• Wipe a dead cat's tail over the eye.
• Hot cow manure placed on a sty will bring it to a head.
• Take a small piece of the skin under an egg shell and apply it to a sty to bring it to a head.
• Rub them with a doorknob which has dew on it.
• Apply the white of chicken manure.

Not to be outdone, the folks in Kentucky have their own special cures.

STYES IN THE EYE: To remove a sty, steal a dish-cloth, rub the sty with it, and bury the dish cloth secretly.

Rub an incipient sty with a plain gold ring warmed by friction with a woolen garment. Pronounce the following couplet:
    'Sty, sty, leave my eye,
    Go to the next passerby.'

If you wear a nutmeg around your neck, you will cure the sty on your eye.

Remove a sty by turning three times on the heel at a cross-roads.
KENTUCKY SUPERSTITIONS, 1920

STY UPON THE EYE-LID: Put a teaspoonful of black tea in a small bag, pour on it enough boiling water to moisten it; then put it on the eye pretty warm. Keep it on all night and in the morning the sty will most likely be gone, if not, a second application is certain to remove it.
DR CHASE'S RECIPES, 1892 EDITION

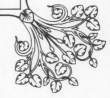

Felon

The word felon *usually brings to mind a wicked person who has committed a crime. But there is another felon, equally as wicked, which attacks fingers and toes. It is a painful abscess found under or near a nail. Felons are sometimes also called whitlow or run-round.*

FELON OR RUN-ROUND ON THE FINGER: Get a toad, split it open, put it on, it will soon begin to stink. Don't take it off till you have another to apply. It will remove the pain and inflammation in a short time.
A NUMBER OF RECEIPTS FOR CURING MAN AND BEAST,
1855

This is obviously one that cures the man and not the beast!

A CHOICE MEDICINE FOR A WHITLOE: Take snail shells and beat the pulpy part of them very well with a convenient quantity of chopped parsley which is to be applied warm to the affected part, and shifted two or three times a day.
THE COMPLETE FAMILY PIECE AND COUNTRY GENTLEMAN AND FARMER'S BEST GUIDE, LONDON 1741

TAK RUSTIE BACON, three snailes, rue, black soap, hony, of each on quantity; first beat the bacon, snailes and rue together, then mingle the hony and black soap and so aplie it.
ENGLISH FOLK REMEDY (DORSET)

It is by poultices, not words, that pain is ended, although pain is by words both eased and diminished.

PETRARCH (1304–74)

Most of the felon remedies are based on the principle of bringing the abscess to a head with the application of some type of poultice. Here are a few choices.

INDIAN TURNIP, BREAD AND MILK: Take either the green or dried root of the Indian turnip which is commonly called jack in the pulpit; grate a teaspoonful into eight tablespoonfuls of sweet milk; simmer for a few minutes; thicken with bread; and apply like a poultice as hot as it can be borne. This is good for both felons and carbuncles.
THE PEOPLE'S HOME MEDICAL BOOK, CLEVELAND, OHIO, 1916

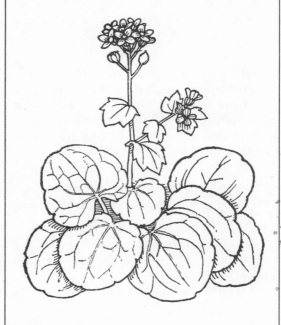

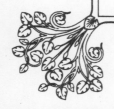
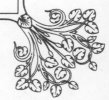

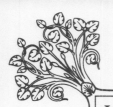

IF RECENT, TO CURE IN SIX HOURS: Venice turpentine, one ounce; and put into it half a teaspoon of water and stir with a rough stick until the mass looks like candied honey, then spread a good coat on a cloth and wrap around the finger. If the case is only recent, it will remove the pain in six hours.
OR
A poultice of clay, from an old log house made and kept wet with spirits of camphor, is also good.
OR
A poke root poultice on a felon, cures by absorption, unless matter is already formed, if it is, it soon brings it to a head, and thus saves much pain and suffering.
DR CHASE'S RECIPES, 1867 EDITION

FELON ON THE HAND: Take of blue-flag root and hellebore equal parts; boil in milk and water; soak the hand in this; as hot as you can bear it, say twenty minutes; then bind the roots on your fingers one hour and a cure will be the result.
LADIES INDISPENSABLE ASSISTANT, NEW YORK, 1851

TOBACCO AND SALT, equal parts, soaked in vinegar. Add a bit of opium. Wrap the tobacco around the sore and keep it wet with the liquid.
UNIDENTIFIED CANADIAN PIONEER'S DIARY

Tobacco was also used in the preparation of an ointment prescribed by Dr Chase. The good doctor left the distinct impression that as far as he was concerned this was one of the few good uses of tobacco.

FELON OINTMENT: Take sweet oil, half a pint and stew a 3 cent plug of tobacco in it until the tobacco is crisped; then squeeze it out and add red lead, one ounce and boil until black; when a little cool, add pulverized camphor gum, one ounce.

Dr Chase went on to note that 'Mrs. Jordan of Clyde, O. paid ten dollars for this recipe and has cured many bad felons, as well as bad fellows with it. Bad fellows because they did not pay her. Certainly this is a rational use of tobacco.'

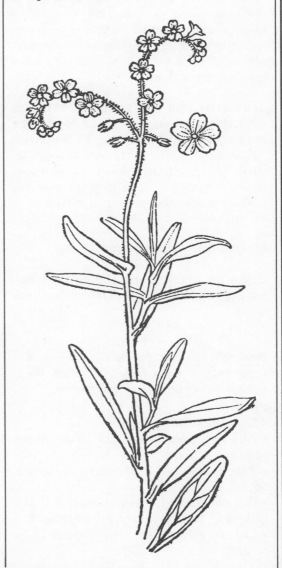

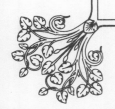

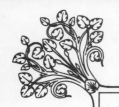
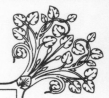

Fevers

And what's a fever but a fit of madness.
SHAKESPEARE, *THE COMEDY OF ERRORS*

TO BREAK A FEVER, catch a grand daddy spider, pull its legs off and swallow it whole and alive.
NORTH CAROLINA FOLK REMEDY.

Although it would appear to be madness to willingly eat a live spider, eating his web is not such a silly idea. Believe it or not, a spider's web contains a powerful fever-reducing agent. And although the next cures also call for live animals, at least you are not required to eat them.

A REMEDY FOR THE FEVER BY THE USE OF WHICH AN OLD LADY OF NOBILITY HAS AIDED MANY PEOPLE: This matron of a noble family cut the ear of a cat, let three drops of the blood fall in some brandy, added a little pepper thereto, and gave it to the patient to drink.
ALBERTUS MAGNUS OR EGYPTIAN SECRETS

No remedy was provided for the cat.

TIE A BAG containing the suffer's nail paring to a live eel. It will carry the fever away.
APPALACHIAN FOLK REMEDY

Naturally, the irrepressible Texans had suggested cures for fever. As usual, the remedies were somewhat...different.

TEXAS REMEDIES
• Boil milkweed and bathe in the water to break a fever.
• Take powdered rattlesnake rattles for ague.
• Put twelve red ants or wood lice in a little bag and tie it around your neck.
• Lie in shallow water near the bank of a river.

• Gather plenty of turds from the wild jack rabbit and dry them in the oven to keep in a jar. When a fever will not totally break, make a very strong tea of the dung and hot water. Strain it and drink it every half hour until the sweating starts. This never fails.

Anyone attempting the next three remedies should remember that walking is not recommended.

PLAISTERS FOR THE FEVER: Beat two handfuls of rue, with as many currants, till they are fine, and well mix'd; spread it on cloths and bind it to the wrists and soles of the feet. This draws from the head; and, if laid on in time, does as much good as pigeons to the feet, in extremity.
A COLLECTION OF RECEIPTS IN COOKERY, PHYSICK AND SURGERY, LONDON 1749.

TO APPEASE THE HEAT OF FEVERS BY AN EXTERNAL REMEDY: Apply to the soles of the feet a mixture or thin cataplasm made of the leaves of tobacco, fit to be cut to fill a pipe with, beaten up with as much of the freshest currants you can get, as will bring the tobacco to the consistence of a poultice.
THE COMPLETE FAMILY PIECE AND COUNTRY GENTLEMAN AND FARMER'S BEST GUIDE, 1741.

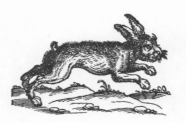

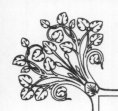

Fever, the eternal reproach to the physicians.
MILTON

PLAISTERS FOR YE FEET: Take a head of garlick and peal it, bruis it and put it into a quarter of a pound of butter and boyl them together well and when cold spread it upon flannell and lay it to ye soles of ye feet. For a fever or vapours approv'd.
THE RECEIPT BOOK OF MRS ANN BLENCOWE, 1694

Many people wrote from Australia telling me they remember wearing a block of camphor around their necks to ward off colds. Here's another reason for walking around smelling funny.

FOR FEVERS: Write upon three almond kernels the following words and take them three mornings in succession:
    Hasta, Hava, Shaver.
Then purchase five cents worth of camphor and make small lozenges from it, and suspend these from your neck. Leave them three days and three nights in that position and remove them at the same hour of the day that they were fastened to your body.
ALBERTUS MAGNUS OR EGYPTIAN SECRETS

Here is one of those complicated recipes which the Lady of the Manor would concoct in her stillroom. Not only did she have to prepare the medicine, she had to cultivate and know when to gather each herb. She was aided by the Gardener's Kalendar *published up until 1775, which gave detailed instructions on the best time to collect each plant for optimum potency.*

SYRUP OF VINEGAR, GOOD TO COOL IN A FEVER: Take a fennel root of a year's growth, four parsley roots of a good bigness; if they are small, take as much as will be equal to the fennel root; and as many succory roots, and two great yellow dock roots: take out the piths of them all, and seethe them in a pottle or gallon of water; add thereto violet leaves, young mallows, and endive, of each a handful, seethe them all, till three pints of their water are consum'd; strain it and let it settle; then take the clearest of this water, and to every quart put a pint of the best white wine vinegar and a pint and half of honey; and seethe and scum it till it comes to be a syrup; put it into a glass, and use it at pleasure; and when you use it, the syrup and borage water, or clean water boil'd of each alike. If you like not honey, put instead thereof one pound of sugar for every pint of honey.
THE ACCOMPLISHED HOUSEWIFE, RECEIPTS IN PHYSICK, 1754

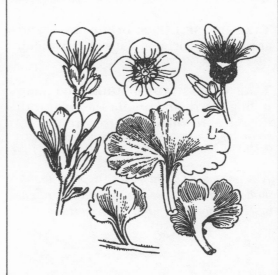

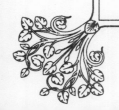
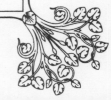

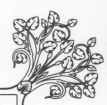

Foot Troubles

And when too short the modish shoes are worn,
You'll judge the seasons by your shooting corns
JOHN GAY, *TRIVIA* (1685-1732)

Centuries ago, modish shoes may have caused many of the fashion-conscious aristocrat's problems with his feet. In most cases, though, the corn sufferer was hobbling around in hand-me-downs, or in more recent times, mail-order shoes. However, the folks in Kentucky had a solution for all shoes— uncomfortably fashionable or plain too small. If at first you filled your shoes with corn and added a little water to it, your shoes would never hurt your feet. But, if you neglected to do this and got a corn, a Kentucky cure was to rub a snail (without its shell) nine times on the corn and then stick the snail on a thorn bush. If a homeless snail is not close at hand,

APPLY SOFT BROWN PAPER moistened with spittle. A few dressings will remove them.
NEW FAMILY RECEIPT BOOK, LONDON, 1815

TAKE HOUSE LEEKS, bruise them and apply to the corns, and it will cure them.
THE FAMILY MAGAZINE, LONDON, 1741

TAKE NIGHTSHADE BERRIES, boil them in hog's lard, and anoint the corn with the salve. It will not fail to cure.
SIX HUNDRED RECEIPTS WORTH THEIR WEIGHT IN GOLD, PHILADELPHIA, 1890

Witches would have a handy supply of nightshade berries because it is a main ingredient in 'flying ointment'. For mere mortals,

A SHAVING OF HARD SOAP will generally draw out a corn in the course of six or eight days. It should be bound on with a rag, changed every day, and the loose skin lightly scraped off.
LYDIA CHILD, THE FAMILY NURSE, BOSTON 1837

APPLY FRESH EVERY MORNING the yeast of small beer, spread on a rag. Or, after paring them closely, apply bruised ivy leaves daily, and fifteen days they will drop out. Tried.
OR, apply chalk, powdered and mixed with water. This also cures warts. Some corns are cured by a pitch plaster.
   All are greatly eased by steeping the feet in hot water wherein oatmeal is boiled. This also helps dry and hot feet.
REVEREND JOHN WESLEY, PRIMITIVE PHYSICK, 1747

A GENTLEMAN IN OHIO offers to pay ten dollars a piece for all corns not cured in three days by binding a bit of cotton batting upon it and wetting it three times a day with spirits of turpentine.
DR CHASE'S RECIPES, 1867 EDITION

Another painful result of badly fitting or new shoes is blisters. Here's advice for relief.

BLISTERS: On the feet, occasioned by walking, are cured by drawing a needle-full of worsted (thread) through them; clip it off at both ends, and leave until the skin peels off.
U.S. PRACTICAL RECEIPT BOOK, 1844

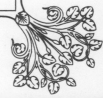

You cannot blame shoes for an ingrown toenail, but it sure makes wearing them painful. So, to get rid of such toenails,

DROP HOT MUTTON TALLOW on the inflamed part.
CANADIAN PIONEER REMEDY

TIE A LIZARD'S LIVER to a leather string around the left ankle. The ingrown toenail should disappear in nine days.
TEXAS REMEDY

Some of our feet troubles are not of our own doing. If you were born pigeon-toed, Mrs. Norma Oram, a great-gran in West Australia, offers this solution.

BUY A PAIR OF SHOES ONE SIZE TOO LARGE and put them on the opposite feet and wear them to bed, thus throwing the feet in the opposite direction. Must be put on every night!

And remember the English proverb,

Wash your hands often, your feet seldom and your head never.

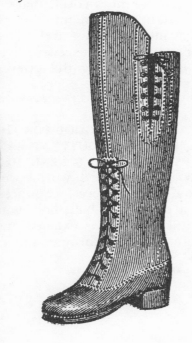

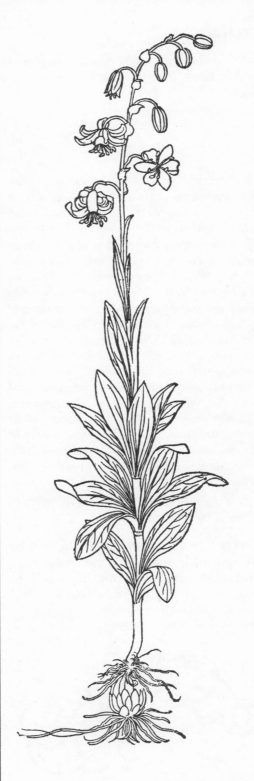

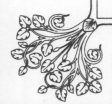

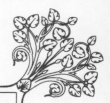

Gout

Gout, unlike any other disease, kills more rich men than poor, more wise men than simple. Great kings, emperors, generals, admirals, and philosophers, have all died of gout.

THOMAS SYDENHAM (1624–89)

The Devils's Dictionary *shares the opinion of Thomas Sydenham and defines gout as 'a physician's name for the rheumatism of a rich patient.' Others contend that the disease only afflicts the wise, citing such gout sufferers as Sir Isaac Newton and Charles Darwin as proof. Still others agree with Sir Richard Blackmore (1650–1729) that 'it is the dissolute and voluptuous Indulgence of sensual Appetites, that administer to the Blood the Seeds of the Gout.' In fact, gout, which is an inflammation of the joints caused by an excess of uric acid in the blood, is not class-conscious and can strike vegetarians and teetotallers just as easily as the hedonist. However, approximately 95 per cent of its victims are male. Since the disease is rare in women and, according to Hippocrates, nonexistent in eunuchs, they can just skip this section.*

Albertus Magnus had a suggestion for warding off gout.

WHEN A PERSON FEELS that he will be smitten with the gout, he must take hold of an anthill and put the same into a bag; cook it and poultice very hot and thus frighten the disease away.
ALBERTUS MAGNUS OR EGYPTIAN SECRETS

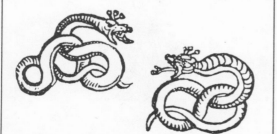

But, if the gout has already claimed you as a victim, here are several ointments and poultices to consider.

FOR ANY HOT SWELLING OR INFLAMATION OF AN OLD SORE OR HOT GOUT: Take ye spawn of frog out of ye clearest water, boyle it while it is a jelly, before it is black, and still it and wash your sores with it a little warm and dip clothes in it and lay it to ye swelling cold.
CURIOUS OLD COOKERY RECEIPTS INCLUDING SIMPLES FOR SIMPLE AILMENTS, LONDON, 1891

TAKE AN OWL, pull off her feathers and pull out her guts; salt her well for a week, then put her into a pot and stop it close, and put her into an oven, that she may be brought into a mummy, which being, beat into a powder and mixed with boar's grease, is an excellent remedy for gout, anointing the grieved place by the fire.
NICHOLAS CULPEPER, *THE ENGLISH PHYSICIAN* 1652

OIL OF EARTHWORMS, GOOD FOR THE JOINTS AND TO EASE GOUTY AND WANDERING PAINS AND TO STRENGTHEN THE NERVES: Take of earth-worms, well washed and cut into pieces, six ounces; oil-olive, a pint and a half; boil them together till the wine is exhaled and lastly strain off the oil through a piece of canvas.
THE FAMILY MAGAZINE, LONDON, 1741

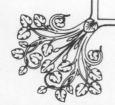
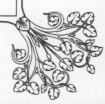

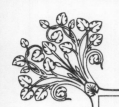

Dear honest Ned is in the gout,
Lies rackt with pain and you without:
How patiently you hear him groan!
How glad the case is not your own!

JONATHAN SWIFT (1667–1745) *ON THE DEATH OF DR. SWIFT*

A GOOD REMEDY FOR GOUT: Take rendered goat's milk, butter, roast cow manure therein, apply to a cloth and put upon the patient's sores.
OR
A SPLENDID AND HITHERTO SECRET FOR THE CURE OF THE SEVEREST PAINS CAUSED BY GOUT, TO EFFECT A CURE IN FIFTEEN MINUTES: After roasting a large and fine orange or lemon upon hot ashes, remove the peelings, pound them with anna flor cassia in a glass mortar and mix it with some breast milk to a poultice. This is an approved remedy and has relieved many persons.
ALBERTUS MAGNUS OR EGYPTIAN SECRETS

AN APPROVED OUTWARD REMEDY FOR THE GOUT: Take the oldest tallow you can get (if it be but a year old, it will do) and garlick, of each equal parts; stamp them together and spread it on canvas, and lay it on. It eases the pain and draws out the humour to admiration.
THE ACCOMPLISHED HOUSEWIFE—RECEIPTS IN PHYSICK, 1754

Reverend Wesley, author of Primitive Physic *and a victim of gout wrote: 'Regard them not who say, the gout ought not to be cured. They mean, it cannot. I know it cannot by their regular prescriptions. But I have known it cured in many cases without any ill effects following.' Here are the methods he used to cure himself.*

THE GOUT IN ANY LIMB: Rub the part with warm treacle and then bind on a flannel smeared therewith. Repeat this if need be, once in twelve hours. This has cured an inveterate gout in thirty-six hours.
OR, drink a pint of strong infusion of elder buds dry or green, morning and evening. This has cured inveterate gout.
OR, at six in the evening, undress and wrap yourself up in blankets; then put your legs up to the knees in water, as hot as you can bear it. As it cools, let hot water be poured in so as to keep you in a strong sweat till ten. Then go to bed well warmed and sweat till morning. I have known this to cure an inveterate gout in a person above sixty who lived eleven years after.
REVEREND JOHN WESLEY, *PRIMITIVE PHYSICK*, 1747

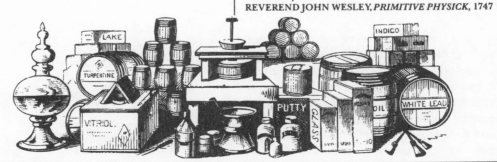

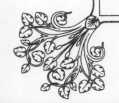
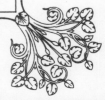

Hayfever

For every ill beneath the sun
There is some remedy or none,
If there be one, resolve to find it;
If not, submit, and never mind it.
ANONYMOUS

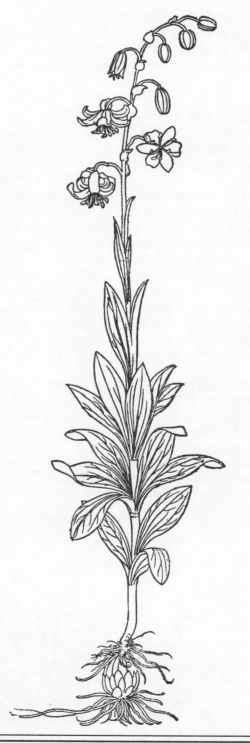

Having suffered from hayfever for years and never having found a satisfactory source of relief, I am reconciled to the advice of the above motto. Perhaps, a fellow sufferer will have better luck with one of these remedies.

SMOKE COFFEE GROUNDS in a pipe and inhale the smoke. Put a green leaf on your forehead until it turns brown.
TEXAS REMEDIES

CUT UP SMALL some of the new hay and make a tea of it. Drink a wineglass of the tea about three times a day and it will relieve and carry off the fever.
THE FARMER'S ADVOCATE, LONDON, ONTARIO, JULY 1883

WHEN THE COMPLAINT first shows itself, try the effect of rest and quiet for a few days, and, if possible, change of air. Keep the bowels gently opened with a saline draught in the mornings and live on a light diet. Take a teaspoonful of Paregoric, or a dose of Kaye's Compound Essence, or any good cough mixture, at bed-time for a few nights. Moisten the nostrils with Eucalyptus, or inhale it in steam.
THE AUSTRALIAN HOUSEHOLD MANUAL, 1899

The last remedy may or may not cure your hayfever but it will certainly play havoc with your bowels. First it calls for a saline draught to keep the bowels open. Then it prescribes paregoric, which, among other things, is a powerful relaxant for spasms of the digestive tract and is still prescribed today for diarrhea. A friend assures me it is very effective.

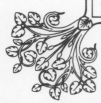

Headaches

'I'm very brave generally,' he went on in a low voice,
'only today I happen to have a headache!'
LEWIS CARROLL, *THE WALRUS AND THE CARPENTER*

Judging by the large number of suggested remedies, headaches were as common throughout the ages as they are today. Lacking aspirins and other so-called wonder-drugs, our forefathers invented an amazing variety of treatments. Some remedies were swallowed, others involved tying substances to the head, some were rubbed on the head, while still others were sniffed. Reverend Wesley offered the whole spectrum.

RUB THE HEAD for a quarter of an hour (Tried)
OR, apply to each temple the thin yellow rind of a lemon newly pared off.
OR, pour upon the palm of the hand a little brandy and some zest of lemon and hold it to the forehead.
OR, a little ether.
OR, if you have caught cold, boil a handful of rosemary, in a quart of water. Put this in a mug, and hold your head (covered with a napkin) over the steam, as hot as you can bear it. Repeat this till the pain ceases (Tried).
OR, snuff up the nose camphorated spirits of lavender.
OR, a little juice of horseradish.
REVEREND JOHN WESLEY, *PRIMITIVE PHYSICK*, 1747

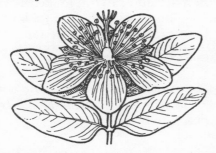

We also owe the expression "Cleanliness is next to Godliness" to the pious Reverend Wesley, who delivered the edict in his sermon 'On Dress'.

The Family Magazine, *published in London in 1741, was promoted as 'Being a Compendious Body of Physick Succinctly Treating of all Diseases and Accidents Incident to Men, Women and Children.' It offered:*

AN EXCELLENT INFUSION FOR MISTS AND CLOUDS OF THE HEAD, VERTIGO, DIZZINESS, HEADACHES ETC.: Take dry peacock's dung (the white part) four ounces; millepedes, alive bruis'd, one ounce, black cherry water, white wine, each one pint and a half: Let them stand cold twenty-four hours; then having clarify'd it, by passing it thro' a flannel bag, add Langius's antepileptick water, three ounces, spirits of lavender compound, one drachm and a half, oil of nutmeg, three drops, syrup of peony compound, six ounces, mix and give a pint nights and morning. [*Millepede goes by the common name of Woodlouse.*]

Jesuit's bark, also known as peruvian or cinchona bark, is most effective in reducing fevers (see Ague and Fever sections). Although either of the following remedies may have been effective for headaches, large or frequent doses could also creat headaches, dizziness and even deafness.

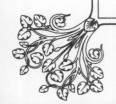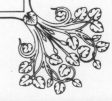

Lord, how my head aches! What a head have I!
It beats as it would fall in twenty pieces.
SHAKESPEARE, *ROMEO AND JULIET*

TO CURE A PAIN OF THE HEAD WHICH RETURNS AT SET TIMES LIKE AN AGUE: Take two scruples of jesuit's bark, make it into a bolus with a sufficient quantity of syrup of gillyflowers. To be repeated every six hours; being constantly taken for three days, it seldom fails of success.
THE COMPLETE FAMILY PIECE AND COUNTRY GENTLEMAN AND FARMER'S BEST GUIDE, 1741

A bolus is a large pill; a scruple is an old measurement used by apothecaries.

MRS. SHERLOCK'S RECEIPT FOR A PAIN IN YE HEAD: two ounces of rhubarb, sliced, one ounce of jesuit's bark in powder, two ounces of sugar candy, two drams of juniper berries, sinamon and nutmeg, of each a dram, a quart of wine infuse it in.
THE RECEIPT BOOK OF MRS ANN BLENCOWE, 1694

It is quite common to find similar remedies in different places. Many European remedies travelled to the New World and Australia. Often, the remedy was changed slightly in its travels.

KENTUCKY REMEDIES:
• You can cure a headache by swallowing a spider's web.
• For headache, bruise a horseradish leaf, wet it and tie it to the head.
• Wear a rattlesnake in the hair day and night to prevent headaches.
• To cure a headache, place the hair that comes from the head in combing under a hidden rock somewhere.

Just east of Kentucky, on the other side of the Appalachian Mountains, people were also hiding their hair under rocks. Only the Appalachian remedy showed more foresight. It suggested that 'when you get your hair cut, gather up on the clippings. Bury them under a rock and you will never have a headache.' (Oldtimers would never allow their hair to be burned or thrown away as it was too valuable.) Those who refused to cut their hair could

BIND WILTED beet leaves on the forehead.
• Tie a flour sack around your head.
• Put several ginseng roots into a piece of brown paper and tie to your head.
• Smear the brow with crushed onions.
• Rub camphor and white whiskey on the head.
APPALACHIAN FOLK REMEDIES

Many remedies call for binding or applying unusual objects to the patient's head. Here are a few more ideas for curative head-gear.

DRY ROSEMARY BEFORE THE FIRE 'till 'twill crumble to a very fine powder one pugil of saffron; and with the powder of rosemary and saffron make the yolk of an egg into a stiff poultis and lay it as hot as you can endure to the temples.
A COLLECTION OF RECEIPTS IN COOKERY, PHYSICK AND SURGERY, LONDON 1749

Pugil is a term of measurement for a handful, or to be more specific, a little handful or a big pinch.

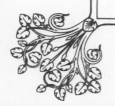
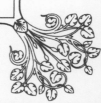

Jack and Jill went up the hill
To fetch a pail of water;
Jack fell down and broke his crown,
And Jill came tumbling after.

Up Jack got and home did trot,
As fast as he could caper,
To old Dame Dob, who patched his nob
With vinegar and brown paper.

FOR MENTAL HEADACHE, coarse brown paper wet with strong cider vinegar will often prove effective and soothing; and sometimes to have the eyes bathed with cool water is a relief to the aching head.
THE HEARTHSTONE, PHILADELPHIA, 1883.

MARIGOLD FLOWERS DISTILLED, GOOD FOR THE PAIN IN THE HEAD: Take Marigold flowers and distill them, then take a fine cloth and wet it in the aforesaid distilled water and so lay it to the forehead of the patient and being so applied, let him sleep if he can; this with God's help will cease the pain.
A QUEEN'S DELIGHT, LONDON, 1671

FOR THE MEGRIME IN THE HEAD: Take goat's dung and mix it with vinegar of squils and anoint the head and temple therewith or this, frankinsence, mirrh and an egg beat them together and apply it to the head and temples.
A BOOK OF SIMPLES, LONDON, C. 1750

Goat's dung seems to be one of the few types of animal manure missed by Martin Luther in this litany.

Tis wonderful how God has put such excellent physic in mere mud; we know that swine's dung stints the blood; horse's serves for the pleurisy, man's heals wounds and black blotches; asses' is used for the bloody flux and cow's with preserved roses serves for epilepsy or for convulsions of children.
MARTIN LUTHER (1483–1546)

This next remedy can be traced back to Nicholas Culpeper who recommended that bayberries 'being made into an electuary with honey, do help the consumption, old coughs, shortness of breathe, and thin rheums as also the megrum.' A megrim is a severe headache on one side of the head only. He also promises 'neither witch or devil, thunder or lightning will hurt a man in a place where the baytree is.'

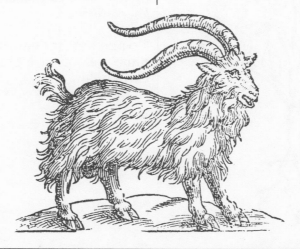

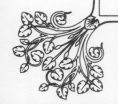

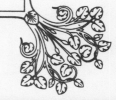

HEADACHE AND CATARRH SNUFF: Take powdered bayberry and snuff it up the nose. It is good for cold in the head, taken on retiring at night.
THE PEOPLE'S MANUAL, WORCESTER, MASSACHUSETTS, 1848

Some people may call the following complaint a 'morning headache'. Others would simply call it a 'hangover'. Whichever, here is an

AMATEUR'S REMEDY FOR MORNING HEADACHE: Take two grains and a half of sulphate of quinine, fifteen drops of laudanum, two tablespoons of simple syrup. Mix and take the whole before your coffee and of course before getting out of bed.
THE FAMILY ORACLE OF HEALTH, ECONOMY, MEDICINE AND GOOD LIVING, LONDON, 1825

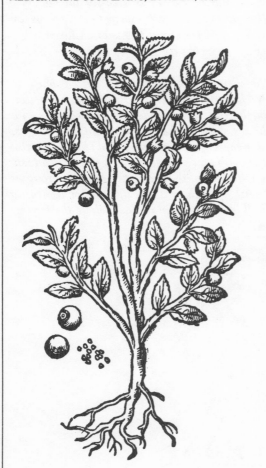

Certainly the ruling tyrant of headaches is the migraine. Contrary to what some people think, the migraine is not a product of the 20th century and its tensions. The migraine headache has been afflicting people throughout history. Samuel Pepys (1633-1703) had a manuscript in his library containing these migraine cures.

FOR THE MIGRAINE A SOVEREIGN MEDICINE: Take three fair sized onions and hollow out the core and save the outer skin, fill the same hole full of black wool and add thereto olive oil and for deficiency thereof other oil and set them in the fire and let them boil and take first one time one of them and hold it in a cloth to your temples and after that the second and when it is cold, take the third until it is cold and it shall be gone forever.
OR
HERE BEGIN GOOD AND TRUE MEDICINE FOR THE MIGRAINE: Take the stem of primrose leaves, two parts and three parts of earth ivy and make juice thereof and take the sick man and lay him upright and put the juice to his nostrils on the contrary side of that where the pain is and do not for anything allow any of the juice to go in his eyes.
STERE ITT WELL

Or, if all other cures have failed, there is one last possibility:

TO RELIEVE HEADACHE IN BED: Discontinue wearing a nightcap and use an extra pillow.
U.S. PRACTICAL RECEIPT BOOK 1844

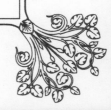

Hiccups

There's often method in the seeming madness of many folk remedies. A popular cure for hiccups is to breathe into a paper bag. In fact, this can be effective since it increases the amount of carbon dioxide inhaled and this gas will control the spasms.

Diversion appears to be the rationale for many of the hiccups cures. By the time you have accomplished the prescribed task, the hiccups will have disappeared, often from lack of attention.

TEXAS REMEDIES:
• Place a damp red thread on a child's forehead, or the head of a burnt match in the child's outer ear, or place a damp nickel on the child's forehead.
• Take a dipper of water from the bucket, close your eyes, take three swallows, open your eyes, look at the bottom of the dipper and then replace the dipper.
• Hold your left elbow for seven minutes.
• Spit on a rock and then turn it over.
• Put a dime in the roof of your mouth and hold it there for thirty minutes.
• Roll a piece of red string into a ball and wet it with saliva. Stick it to your forehead just above the eyes and look at it.
• Tighten a belt around your chest.

PLACING FINGERS TOGETHER: Without leaning on anything, see how nearly together you can keep the ends of the small fingers being very careful never to allow them to touch.
THE PEOPLE'S HOME MEDICAL BOOK, CLEVELAND, OHIO, 1916

YOU CAN CURE HICCOUGHS if you put the ends of both thumbs behind the ears and push inward.

If you have a hiccough, think of your lover. If he loves you, you will not have it anymore.
KENTUCKY SUPERSTITIONS, 1920

Try reciting this old English verse along with the next two cures.

Hickup, snickup, stand up, straight up, One drop, two drops—good for the hick-up.

THE BEST REMEDY in ordinary hiccoughs is about twenty-five grains of common table salt placed in the mouth and swallowed with a sip of water.
THE HEARTHSTONE, PHILADELPHIA 1883

TAKE A DRAUGHT OF COLD WATER and rub the breast and stomach with pepper and vinegar.
FARMER'S DIRECTORY AND HOUSEKEEPER'S ASSISTANT, TORONTO, 1851

Hippocrates said that sneezing will stop a hiccup. Nearly twenty-two hundred years later, Reverend Wesley gave the same advice along with some other suggestions.

HICKUP, TO CURE: Swallow a mouthful of water, stopping the mouth and the ears. (Tried)
OR, three drops of oil of cinnamon on a lump of sugar (Tried).
OR, two or three preserved damsons.
OR, ten drops of chemical oil of amber dropped on sugar and then mixed with a little water.

HICKUP, TO PREVENT: Infuse a scruple of musk in a quart of mountain wine and take a small glass every morning.
REVEREND JOHN WESLEY, *PRIMITIVE PHYSICK*, 1747

Musk originally referred to an odoriferous substance secreted in the male musk-deer, native to central Asia. It was used as the basis of perfumes and in some medicines as a stimulant or antispasmodic. Gradually the term came to apply to the secretions of a number of animals like the muskrat and musk-ox that had a musky odour. Since the 17th century, musk scent similar to the secretions of the musk-deer has been artificially made.

A POWDER TO STOP THE HICKUP IN MAN, WOMAN OR CHILD: Put as much dillseed, finely powder'd as will lie on a shilling, into two spoonsful of black cherries, and take it presently.
A COLLECTION OF RECEIPTS IN COOKERY, PHYSICK AND SURGERY, LONDON, 1749

Nicholas Culpeper also recommended dill seed for hiccups. 'It stayeth the hiccough, being boiled in wine, but smelled unto, being tied in a bag.'

If you can perform the next feat, you really deserve to be cured: repeat the following verse three times in one breath.

When a twister twisting, twists him a twist,
For twisting a twist three twists he must twist;
But if one of the twists untwists from the
  twist,
The twist untwisting untwists all the twist.
ENGLISH NURSERY CHARM FOR CURING HICCOUGHS

If you do it successfully, even while hiccupping, you might also consider going into business making hard-sell commercials for radio and television.

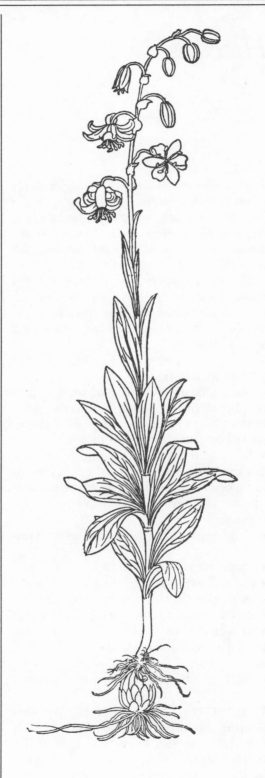

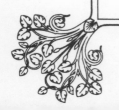
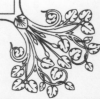

Hysterics

Idleness begets ennui, ennui the hypochondriac, and that a diseased body. No laborius person was ever yet hysterical.
THOMAS JEFFERSON, 28 MARCH 1787

The work involved in preparing many of these remedies would surely solve any problems begotten by idleness.

FOR THE HYSTERICKS OR NERVOUS COMPLAINT: Take hysop, skunk cabbage root, and Solomon seal root, equal part, make a strong syrup, to which add a little ginger, as this last is good for wind. Take a draught of this every morning as soon as out of bed, another on going to bed, and you will soon begin to mend.
THE FAMILY PHYSICIAN AND THE FARMER'S COMPANION, SYRACUSE, NEW YORK, 1840

This is a quick remedy, if you happen to have powdered chicken manure on hand.

TAKE DRIED CHICKEN MANURE, grind it to powder and give a pinch of it to the patient in a prune. It is a quick remedy.
ALBERTUS MAGNUS OR EGYPTIAN SECRETS

VAPORS AND FAINTING SPELLS: Burning a lock of the victim's hair in a shovel held beneath the nose is supposed to be very effective; or, simply burn a feather beneath the victim's nose.
TENNESSEE FOLK REMEDIES

Although these particular Tennessee remedies do not require a spoon, I should mention the Tennessee rule that medicine is always administered in a silver spoon.

HYSTERICS ACCOMPANIED BY FAINTING: Take the warts commonly growing on the shanks of steers, cut them fine, dry them in an iron pan over a glowing flame until they become yellowish, bruise them gently and give of this powder as much as the point of a table-knife will hold, in wine or other liquor, to the patient, who must keep herself warm.
ALBERTUS MAGNUS OR EGYPTIAN SECRETS

Apparently only women suffered from hypochondria, vapours, nervous complaints and hysterics. For virgins there was an obvious cure.

I advise maidens who suffer from hysteria to marry as soon as possible. For if they conceive, they will be cured.
HIPPOCRATES, *ABOUT MAIDENS* (460–377 B.C.)

GET A LITTLE ANTIMONIAL WINE down the throat, so as to cause vomiting; this puts an end to the fits. A purge should be taken, as soon as the emetic has operated, and the feet bathed in warm water—The cold bath is the best preventative to this complaint.
THE HOUSEKEEPER'S ALMANAC, NEW YORK, 1842

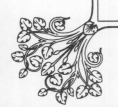
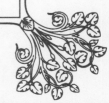

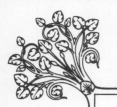

Indigestion

(Also see Stomach troubles and Colic)

Indigestion is—that inward fate
Which makes all Styx through one small liver flow
LORD BYRON (1788–1824), *DON JUAN*

Some call it dyspepsia, acid stomach, indigestion, flatulence or heartburn, but whatever it is called, it is unpleasant. One French writer has called dyspepsia 'remorse of a guilty stomach.' When a certain Dr Abernethy was asked how to cure dyspepsia, he replied: 'Live upon sixpence and earn it.' If that seems a little severe, there are other suggestions.

CURE FOR INDIGESTION: Rise early and walk a mile before breakfast, then drink a cupful of cold spring water—half a pint will not be too much if the stomach is strong enough—and walk another mile. Continue this treatment regularily for a month or six weeks.
THE PEOPLE'S ALMANAC, MONTREAL, 1855

TAKE THREE BLACK PEPPER CORNS every morning before breakfast.
REMEDY FROM DIARY OF A CANADIAN PIONEER

FOR SOME FORMS OF DYSPEPSIA, there is no more simple and effective remedy than raw cranberries. Carry a supply in pocket and eat them frequently during the day. They will cure headaches as well.
THE NEW COOK BOOK, TORONTO, 1906

DYSPEPSIA: See that you have a good laugh once a day. A really good laugh exercises the diaphram, expands the lungs, shakes up the liver, benefits the heart and practically every gland and organ in the body.
ANONYMOUS

The Irish also have a proverb: 'A good laugh and a long sleep are the best cures in the doctor's book.'

Heartburn comes when you've eaten too much of what you shouldn't and there is excessive acidity of the gastric juices. So, the inclusion of alkaline substances in the following recipes makes good sense.

TWO TABLESPOONS OF CARBONATE OF SODA to one teaspoon of ground ginger mixed. Take one teaspoonful in hot water before breakfast.
THE AUSTRALIAN COUNTRY WOMEN'S
ASSOCIATION, 1937

Ginger, along with peppermint, is one of the best loved and used spices. It helps to stop griping pains in flatulence.

TO CURE HEARTBURN: A teacup full of chamomile tea, or a small quantity of chalk scrapped into a glass of water, are deemed effectual remedies.
THE COMPLEAT VERMIN KILLER AND USEFUL POCKET COMPANION, DUBLIN, 1778.

ACID STOMACH: Take good unslaked lime, the quarter of the size of a hen's egg, to one pint of soft water, strain, keep cool, take one teaspoonful to half a teacupful of new milk, night and morning. Infallible.
A NUMBER OF RECEIPTS FOR CURING MAN AND BEAST, 1855.

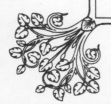
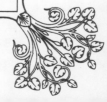

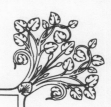

Dyspepsy is the ruin of most things;
empires, expeditions, and everything else.
THOMAS DE QUINSEY (1785–1859)

THE HEARTBURNING: Drink a pint of cold water.

OR, drink slowly a decoction of camomile flowers.

OR, eat four or five oysters.

OR, chew five or six peppercorns a little; then swallow them.

OR, chew fennel or parsley and swallow your spittle.

OR, a piece of spanish liquorice.

REVEREND JOHN WESLEY, *PRIMITIVE PHYSICK*, 1747

AN INFALLIBLE POWDER FOR THE HEARTBURN AND SWOONING FITS: Take the whitest chalk, six ounces; crabs-eyes, crabs-claws, of each one ounce and a half; treble refin'd sugar, half an ounce; oil of nutmegs, six drops: mix and make a powder, adding to it fine bole six drams. Give the patient one drachm in the morning fasting and at night going to bed for a fortnight together, taking a gentle purge once in six days to carry it off.
THE FAMILY MAGAZINE, LONDON, 1741.

FOR THE HEART-ACHE OR HEARTBURN: For the one, keep a conscience void of offense*, for the other chew magnesia or chalk, or drink a tumbler of cold milk.
THE IMPROVED HOUSEWIFE, HARTFORD, 1846

The Improved Housewife added this rather bitter footnote: 'The remedy cannot apply where the wife has a drunken husband.'

Science has confirmed Reverend Wesley's last suggestion. During the Second World War, a substance in licorice was discovered to be extremely beneficial in helping to heal gastric ulcers.

Finally, for those who want to throw caution to the wind, a word from Mark Twain.

Part of the secret of success in life is to eat what you like and let the food fight it out inside.

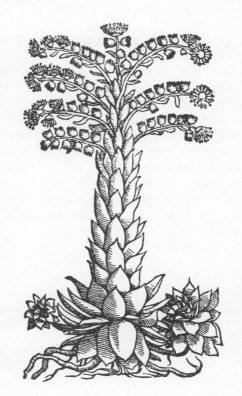

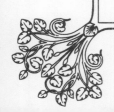
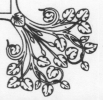

Insomnia

Early to bed and early to rise,
Makes a man healthy, wealthy and wise.
BENJAMIN FRANKLIN, *POOR RICHARD'S ALMANACK*, 1735

There's an English proverb which says: 'Six hours sleep for a man, seven for a woman and eight for a fool.' But, even a fool is better off than someone with no sleep at all. If you're an insomniac and have counted enough sheep to populate the whole continent of Australia, perhaps you should try one of these.

TO FACILITATE HEALTHY SLEEP: Procure two rabbit ears, place them under the pillow of a person who cannot sleep, without his knowledge.
ALBERTÚS MAGNUS OR EGYPTIAN SECRETS

A CORDIAL TO PROCURE SLEEP AND REST: Take a quart of the best unsophisticated claret wine; put into it a handful of cowslip flowers; one handful of borage flowers and a slip of rosemary, set it on the fire and when it is ready to burn, smother it in the first flame and keep it in the pot till it is cold, then strain it and put thereto three ounces of clove gillyflowers well mingled together and every night at your going to bed, take a wineglassful of it, you must not warm it a second time.
THE TRUE PRESERVER, 1682

HOW TO MAKE A TEA FOR A SLEEPLESS PERSON: Make a tea of Jerusalem Oak which only grows in the woods, and drink it, as you would any other tea, before going to bed.
SIX HUNDRED RECEIPTS WORTH THEIR WEIGHT IN GOLD, PHILADELPHIA, 1890

Jerusalem oak is none other than ragweed, a noxious herb to which many people are allergic.

TAKE A WARM BATH ten minutes before lying down, or use the fleshbrush for a quarter of an hour. If you do not feel disposed to sleep, commence counting one thousand; before you get to five hundred, you will most probably fall asleep.
U.S. PRACTICAL RECEIPT BOOK, 1844

A flesh brush is just that—a brush used for rubbing the flesh to promote good circulation. The Porter Health Almanac *for 1832 explained its virtues: 'The use of a flesh brush is an exercise in promoting a full and free perspiration and circulation. Almost everyone knows what good currying will do for horses in making them sleek and gay, lively and active; even so much as to be worth half the feeding.' Perhaps it would be wiser to curry yourself in the morning rather than to lie in bed feeling gay, lively and active.*

Sleep is a priceless treasure; the more one has of it, the better it is.
CHINESE PROVERB

The theory behind the following seems to be that nice odours are conducive to sleep.

TO PROCURE SLEEP: Wash the head in a decoction of dill seed, and smell it frequently.
LADIES INDISPENSABLE ASSISTANT, NEW YORK 1851

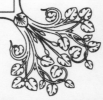

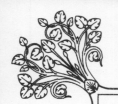

Sleep vanishes before the house of care.
TIBULLUS (54–18 B.C.)

TO SECURE NATURAL SLEEP AND REST: Take oil of mace and rose salve, of one as much as of the other: Mix well together; with this anoint the temples, the neck, the nostrils, the pulses of both arms, and the soles of the feet. Repeat this several days in succession before retiring to bed. It brings on natural sleep.
ALBERTUS MAGNUS OR EGYPTIAN SECRETS

IF A MAN CANNOT SLEEP, take henbane seed and juice of garden mint: Stir together. Smear the head therewith. He will be better.
LACNUNGA, 10TH C. EARLY ANGLO-SAXON REMEDY

Mint was believed to repel vermin and was often scattered around the bed along with other strewing herbs such as rue, wormwood, sage and chamomile to protect against disease. Those who could not blame bedbugs for their sleepless nights were offered this next remedy. I would definitely only advise trying it if you sleep alone.

SLEEPLESSNESS, SIMPLE REMEDY, BUT SUCCESSFUL WITH MANY: For those troubled with sleeplessness from literary labours or other disturbances of the nervous system, a writer of experience says, "just before retiring eat two or three raw onions with a little bread, lightly spread with fresh butter, which will produce the desired effect, saving the stupefying action of drugs."
DR CHASE'S RECIPES, 1892 EDITION

Unlike his modern counterparts, Dr Chase refused to recommend drugs.

INSOMNIA: Take a grain or two of camphor at bed-time. This is surer and safer than laudanum.
THE HOUSEKEEPER'S ALMANAC, NEW YORK, 1842

But not everyone agrees with avoiding drugs, Here's a cynic's approach to the problem.

Slumber, which has been glorified by every poet, isn't above a little bribe of two sleeping tablets.
ANONYMOUS

Many a good night of rest has been ruined by nightmares. So, it is best to take measures to prevent them.

IF YOU GO TO SLEEP on the flat of the back, you will not have a nightmare. A cure for the nightmare is found by turning the shoes upside down with the toes towards the head of the bed.
KENTUCKY SUPERSTITIONS, 1920

TO PREVENT NIGHT MARE: Avoid heavy suppers, and on going to bed take the following mixture. Sal-volatile, twenty drops, tincture of ginger, two drachms.
THE FAMILY MANUAL, NEW YORK 1845

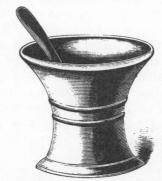

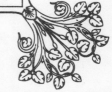

Jaundice

All looks yellow to the jaundic'd eye
ALEXANDER POPE (1688-1744)

A number of these remedies were probably successful because the patient paled just at the thought of having to take any of these potions.

MRS. SKILLIN'S RECEIPT FOR THE YELLOW JAUNDICE: Take a pint of strong beer or ale, nine earthwormes. Slit them and scoure them from their slime, then take a handful of sallendine and one pennyworth of saffron and put all these together and let them boyle up once or twice, then let them stand till they are cold, then strain out and drink this three mornings.
A BOOK OF SIMPLES, 1750

A GREAT ARCANUM AGAINST THE JAUNDICE: Take troches of vipers (or rather viper's flesh dry'd) fifteen grains, salt of amber, three grains; saffron, two grains, make a powder.
OR
DR. WILLIS'S PRESCRIPTION FOR THE JAUNDICE: Take the roots of the greater nettles, a pound; saffron, a scruple: bruise them well, and extract a tincture with white wine. Take three ounces in the morning for four or five days.
THE FAMILY MAGAZINE, LONDON, 1741

DRINK FOR JAUNDICE: Tie up soot and saffron, equal parts, in a clothe to the size of half a hen's egg; let it lie in a glass of water overnight; in the morning put the yolk of an egg, beaten into this water and drink it. Do this three mornings, skipping three until nine doses have been taken.
DR CHASE'S RECIPES, 1867 EDITION

As you may have noticed, most of these remedies include saffron as one of the ingredients. The spice is grown in the Mediterranean region and has been used for thousands of years, since biblical times. It takes the pistils of some four thousand crocus flowers to make a single ounce of saffron. For this reason, it has been one of the more expensive spices.

The use of saffron in jaundice remedies is an example of the practice of the Doctrine of Signatures, or the belief in healing by similarities. It was thought that nature had indicated the uses of plants for medicinal purposes by their appearance, colour or smell. The yellow color of saffron was a sign from God that it should be used to cure the yellowish victim.

As always, people read the signs of nature in different ways. I can assure you of the outcome of the next remedy—husking walnuts will turn the hands a warm brown colour that will remain long after the jaundice has gone.

FOR THE JAUNDICE: To four pounds of the husks of wallnuts, put half a pound of wormseed and as much flower of brimstone. Draw it off in a cold still and let a tea cupfull be taken every morning for a month. This is an excellent medicine for jaundice and hath done great cures.
OLD ENGLISH REMEDY

DRINK PLENTIFULLY of Decoction of Carrots.
CANADIAN PIONEER REMEDY

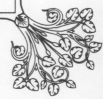

Jaundice is the disease that your friends diagnose.
SIR WILLIAM OSLER (1849-1919)

While amateur diagnosis might be easy, most of the old medicines were pretty hard to force down anyone's throat. So, I would lay odds that given the choice, most people would haved opted for these next two remedies to cure their jaundice.

HOW TO CURE THE YELLOW JAUNDICE WITHOUT MEDICINE, OR GIVING ANYTHING TO THE PATIENT WHATSOEVER: Take the patient's morning urine and put the same into a bottle; then take a piece of saffron and tie it up in a fine piece of muslin, and put the same in the bottle amongst the said urine; and only desire the patient wholly to abstain from drinking either milk or malt liquor for one month, proved a great number of times. This prescription is worth more money than the price of this book.
DR PARKINS THE FAMILY PHYSICIAN, 1814

We do not know how much Dr Parkins, who modestly subtitled his adaptation of Culpeper's Herbal 'The Holy Temple of Wisdom,' was charging for his book.

FOR JAUNDICE catch about a half dozen 'old sows' (Gray hearth bugs) and boil them in water. Then stir into the mixture enough meal to make a cake. Place it on a chimney piece. When the cake is done, the person will be well.
KENTUCKY SUPERSTITIONS 1920

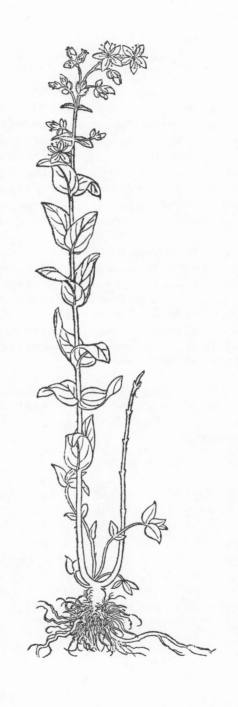

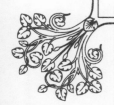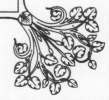

Lockjaw

Lockjaw is the popular name for tetanus—once a dreaded infectious disease. The common name describes the jaw spasms and difficulty victims experience in opening their mouths. Tetanus germs exist in all kinds of dirt and rust and can infect open wounds or punctures. Today injections are used to prevent this sometimes fatal disease. In the past people had to rely on treatments such as these.

TO RELIEVE AND PREVENT: The following remedy, simple as it is, is said to have saved thousands from death by lockjaw. Smoke the wound or bruise with the smoke of wool. Twenty minutes in the smoke of wool, will allay the worst case of inflammation arising from a wound.
DR CHASE'S RECIPES, 1892 EDITION

A RIND OF PORK bound on a wound occasioned by a needle, pen or nail, prevents the lockjaw. It should always be applied.
THE LADY'S ANNUAL REGISTER AND HOUSEWIFE'S MEMORANDUM BOOK, BOSTON, 1838

PUT HOT WOOD ASHES into hot water, wet thick clothes in the water, apply to the jaws as quickly as possible and at the same time bathe the entire backbone with hot vinegar with either cayenne or mustard added. If vinegar is not at hand, use hot water in its place. Persist in this treatment and the jaws will relax.
THE PEOPLE'S HOME MEDICAL BOOK, CLEVELAND, OHIO 1916

IT SHOULD BE BORNE IN MIND that almost any wound may cause lockjaw, as it is caused by a germ; therefore the safest remedy in all cases is to apply warm turpentine at once, and keep the wound covered.
THE AUSTRALIAN HOUSEHOLD MANUAL, 1899

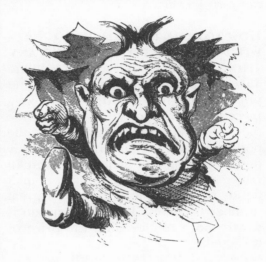

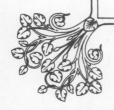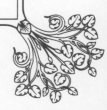

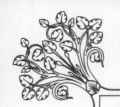

Love Troubles

O ye gods, have ye ordained for every malady a medicine, for every sore a salve, for every pain a plaister, leaving only love remedyless.

JOHN LYLY (1554-1606)

Mr Lyly could not have been looking in the right books. There were a number of remedies for various love maladies around in his day, many of them attributed to Albertus Magnus. In medieval times, marriages among the nobility and much of the small but growing middle-class were arranged for reasons of money, extending land holdings or forging alliances. That created a problem for the husbands.

HOW TO CAUSE YOUR INTENDED WIFE TO LOVE YOU: Take feathers from a rooster's tail, press them three times into her hand. Probatum. Or, take a turtle dove into your mouth, talk to your friend agreeably, kiss her and she will love you so dearly that she cannot love another.
ALBERTUS MAGNUS OR EGYPTIAN SECRETS

Another problem was that spouses often knew little about each other, sometimes meeting for the first time on their wedding night.

TO TRY IF A PERSON IS CHASTE: Sap of raddish squeezed into the hand will prove what you want to know. If they do not fumble or grabble, they are all right.
ALBERTUS MAGNUS OR EGYPTIAN SECRETS

The book Egyptian Secrets *has several remedies for various love problems. However, it is very unlikely these cures come from the real Albertus Magnus (1206-80). This German was one of the most learned men of his time and the famous teacher of St. Thomas Aquinas. He knew all of Aristotle's works and was one of the most eminent naturalists of his day. And because of his widely acknowledged intellect, several people used his name for their own books. One of the most famous forgeries was a book of "Secrets" concerning medicine that was actually written by one of his own pupils. Quite likely* Egyptian Secrets *was originally written by a student of Magnus, although a number of people have modified and added or even published their own* Egyptian Secrets *through the centuries. So the true origin of these cures is anyone's guess.*

TO RESTORE MANHOOD: Buy a pike as they are sold in the fish market, carry it noiselessly to a running water, there let whale oil run into the snout of the fish, throw the fish into the running water and then walk stream upward, and you will recover your strength and former powers.
EGYPTIAN SECRETS

ANOTHER REMEDY TO RESTORE MANHOOD: Take a new fresh laid egg, if possible, one that is yet warm. Pour whale oil over it and boil the egg in it; the oil then should be poured into a running water, stream downward, never stream upward, then open the egg a little, carry it to an ant's hill, of the large red specie, as are found in fir tree forests and there bury the egg. As soon as the ants have devoured the egg, the weak and troubled person will be restored to former strength and vigour.
EGYPTIAN SECRETS

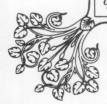
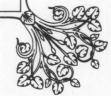

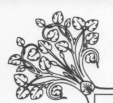

Courtly love was a very popular concept in the Middle Ages. The problem was that sometimes this ritualistic wooing got out of hand.

A MAGIC FOR ONE WHO HAS BEEN INFATUATED BY ILLICIT LOVE TO A FEMALE: Such a person must put a pair of shoes on, and walk therein until his feet perspire, but must walk fast, so that the feet do not smell badly; then take off the right shoe, drink some beer or wine out of this shoe, and he will from that moment lose all affection for her.
OR
When you are infatuated and bewitched by a woman so that you may not love nay other, then take blood of a buck and grease your head therewith and you will soon be all right again.
EGYPTIAN SECRETS

You may have noticed that all these love-lorn remedies are for men. Women may have represented the knightly ideal of goodness, but in truth they were second-class citizens during the Middle Ages in religion, society and the law. So it is not surprising that they were ignored by the medical writers, who were usually men. However, there was one area of love remedies that applied equally to both sexes—aphrodisiacs.

TAKE THE LIVER OF A SPARROW, a pigeon's heart, a hare's kidney, a swallow's womb, and dry and crush them into a powder. Add an equal weight of your own blood. For an infallible potion, dry off the whole and add the resultant powder to a soup.
EGYPTIAN SECRETS

TAKE THE STONE CALLED CHALCEDONY. It is black or red, and may be found in the stomachs of swallows. Wrap the stone in a piece of soft calf skin and wear it under the left armpit.
EGYPTIAN SECRETS

This next recipe for an aphrodisiac in the form of a pie comes from Cartoleomeo Scappi, the private chef to His Holiness Pope Pius V!

TO MAKE A PIE OF BULL'S TESTICLES, take four of them and boil them in water and salt. Cut them in slices, sprinkle them with white pepper, salt, cinnamon and nutmeg. Prepare separately a mince of lamb's kidney, gravy, three slices of lean ham, a good pinch of chopped marjoram, thyme and three cloves. Prepare the pastry for the pie. Then begin to make a layer on your pie dish with the ham, then a layer of slices of testicles, sprinkle well with the mince and so on. Before shutting the pie, add a glass of wine. Put in the oven and serve hot.

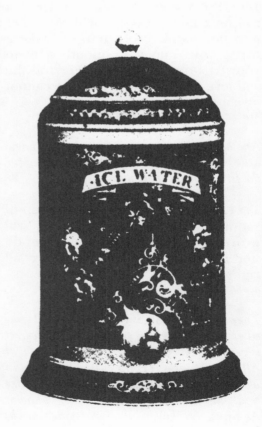

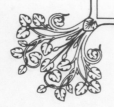
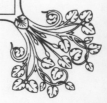

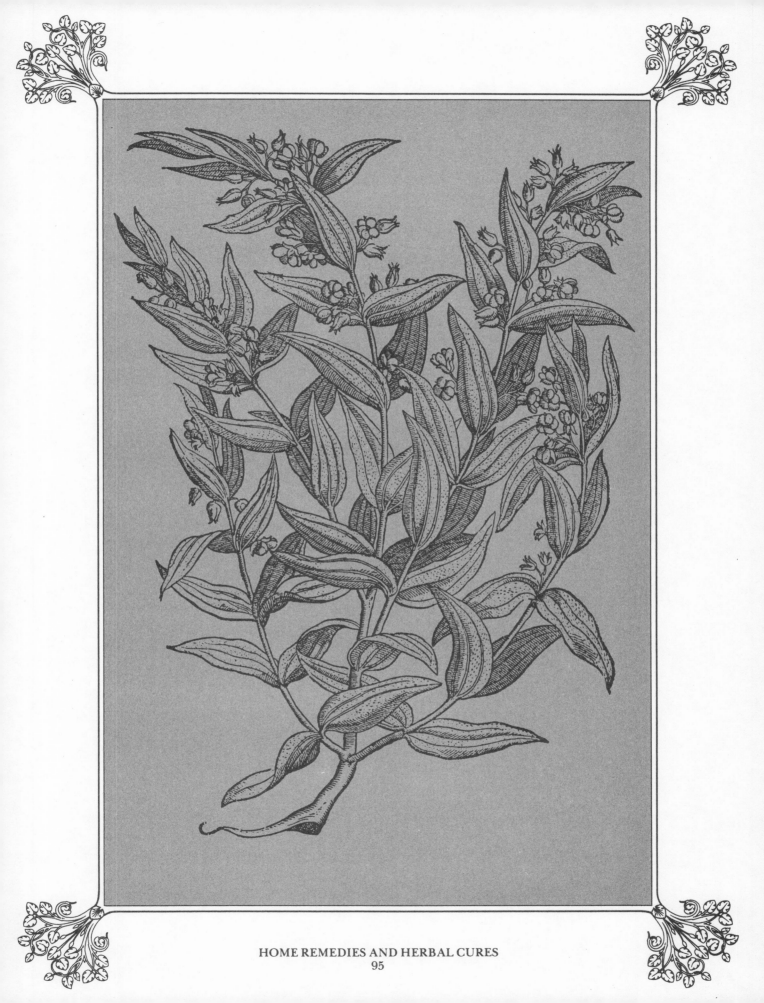

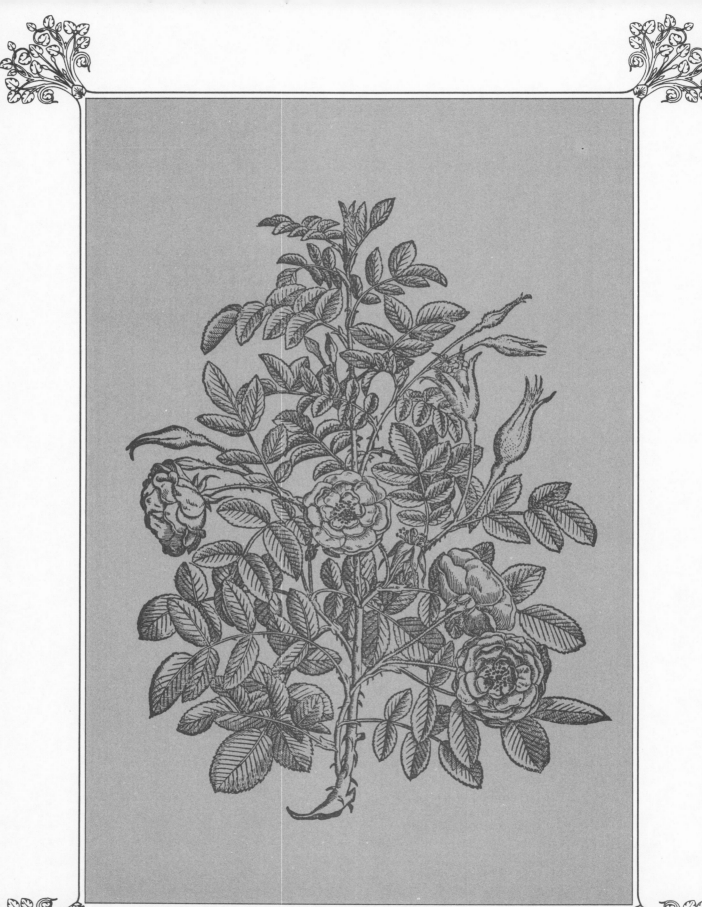

Quinsy

O that I now were changed into a quinsy,
To seize her throat, and strangle the evil jade.
PLAUTUS (254–184 BC)

Quinsy is the old-fashioned term for a bad case of tonsillitis, where the tonsils become abscessed. According to Dr Chase, 'This disease occurs principally in spring and autumn when vicissitudes of heat and cold are frequent. It affects especially the young and sanguine, and a disposition to it is often acquired by frequent attacks. It commences with an unusual sense of tightness in the throat, particularly on swallowing which is often effected with difficult and pain. The inflammation generally attacks one tonsil first, which, in a day or two it sometimes leaves and effects the other, and not unfrequently quits them both suddenly and flies to the lungs.' Of course, he provided several cures.

TO CURE QUINSY: Roast three or four large onions. Peel them quickly and beat them flat with a rolling-pin. Immediately place them in a thin muslin bag that will reach from ear to ear and about three inches deep. Apply it speedily as warm as possible to the throat. Keep it on day and night, changing it when the strength of the onions appears to be exhausted and substituting fresh ones. Flannel must be worn round the neck after the poultice is removed.
OR
Apply a large white bread toast half an inch thick, dipped in brandy to the crown of the head till it dries; or, swallow slowly white rose water mixed with syrup of mulberries; or draw in as hot as you can, for ten or twelve minutes together, the fumes of red rose leaves, or camomile flowers, boiled in water and vinegar, or of a decoction of bruised hemp seed. This speedily cures the sore throat, peripneumony and inflammation of the uvula.
DR CHASE'S RECIPES, 1880 EDITION

Never in the history of medicine have so many physicians owed so much economic security to a single operation as to tonsillectomy.

QUOTED FROM NEW YORK TIMES MAGAZINE BY LYMAN RICHARDS, 1953

A CURE FOR QUINSY: If it rages very bad, bleed under the tongue, otherwise omit. Take good vinegar, two quarts, heat it in a coffee pot, take the snout into your mouth and steam your throat as hot as you can bear it; wet flannel in vinegar and put it around your neck; continue this process for twelve hours with intermissions for rest. I have tried this method on myself, and many others, and have never known it fail.
THE FAMILY PHYSICIAN AND FARMER'S COMPANION, SYRACUSE, NEW YORK, 1840

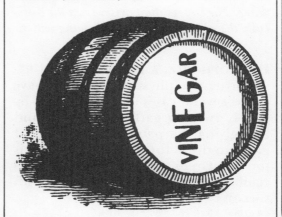

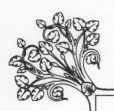

Rabies

Five centuries ago, in a work entitled a Papal Garland Concerning Poisons, William de Marra attempted to answer that puzzling question of why dogs are more prone to rabies than other animals. His answer: the dog, living so close to human beings, is more provoked to wrath and sadness than other animals. The folklore and superstitions concerning rabies date from the time of the ancient Greeks. Each society had its own cures for people bitten by rabid dogs, but none was as drastic as that of the Danes who simply strangled the victims straightoff to save them from the slow, agonizing death. In Kentucky, the opposite view was held.

THE HAIR OF A DOG is good for its bite. If a dog that bites a person goes mad after, so will the person. Therefore kill the dog straightway.
KENTUCKY SUPERSTITIONS, 1920

Rabies was often called hydrophobia because of the misconception that it caused a fear of water. In fact, rabies, which slowly attacks the central nervous system, does no such thing. The superstition arises from the difficulty the victims have in swallowing water.

HYDROPHOBIA, A PORTUGUESE CURE: A Portuguese physician claims to have cured several cases of hydrophobia by simply rubbing garlic into the wound and giving the patient a decoction of garlic to drink for several days. This is the old Greek treatment, which, it is claimed, was practised by them with success.
DR CHASE'S RECIPES, 1892 EDITION

AT UDINA, in Friule, a poor man lying under the frightful tortures of hydrophobia, was cured with some draughts of vinegar, given him by mistake, instead of another potion. A physician at Padua got intelligence of this event at Udina and tried the same remedy upon a patient in the hospital, administering to him a pound of vinegar in the morning, another at noon and a third at sunset, and the man was speedily and perfectly cured.
THE HOUSEHOLD BOOK OF PRACTICAL RECEIPTS, LONDON, 1871

Was he cured—or pickled?

GRECIAN REMEDY: Eat the green shoots of asparagus raw, sleep and perspiration will be induced, and the disease can be thus cured in any stage of canine madness.
OR
A QUAKER REMEDY—FIFTY YEARS SUCCESSFUL: The dried root of elecampane; pulverize it and measure out nine heaping tablespoons and mix it with two or three teaspoonfuls of pulverized gum arabic; then divide it into nine equal portions. When a person is biten by a rabid animal take one of these portions and steep it in one pint of new milk until nearly half the quantity of milk is evaporated; then strain and drink it in the morning, fasting for four or five hours after. The same dose is to be repeated three mornings in succession, then skip three, and so on until the nine doses are taken.
DR CHASE'S RECIPES, 1867 EDITION.

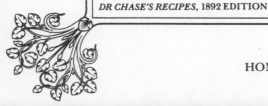

I found this yellowed old newspaper clipping in a scrapbook of medical recipes carefully cut out and saved by a Canadian pioneer.

A GERMAN FOREST-KEEPER, eighty-two years old, not wishing to carry to the grave with him an important secret, has published a recipe he has used for fifty years, and which he says, has saved several men and a great number of animals from a horrible death by hydrophobia. The bite must be bathed as soon as possible with warm vinegar water, and, when this has dried, a few drops of muriatic acid poured upon the wound will destory the poison of the saliva and relieve the patient from all present and future danger.

The English had a preventive for rabies. Any dog that howled on Christmas Eve was often immediately killed because it was believed that it would most certainly go mad before the year was out. If any dog escaped detection, the English tried to save the victim's life with one of these.

A CURE FOR THE BITE OF A MAD DOG: Write on a piece of paper these words, Rebus, Rebus, Epitepscum; give it to the Party or Beast bitten to eat in bread. This never fails.
THE COMPLEAT HOUSEWOMAN, 1711

FOR ANY CREATURE BITT BY A MAD DOG: Take the quantity of five great primrose roots and some leaves; some box leaves, but not so much as the other; a little barke of golden withey or willow, wash them and pound them into a Quart of black cow's milk and let them stand all night together.
FROM A PLAIN PLANTAIN, A 17TH C. HOUSEHOLD RECEIPT BOOK

TAKE FOUR OUNCES OF RUE, four ounces of London Treacle, four spoonfuls of scrap'd Pewter, and four ounces of Garlick; stamp the Garlick, and boil all in a pottle of stale strong Ale; strain this drink; let that which is thick be apply'd to the wound, and take nine spoonfuls of the clear for nine days altogether.
A COLLECTION OF RECEIPTS IN COOKERY, PHYSICK AND SURGERY, LONDON, 1749

A MEDICINE FOR ANYONE THAT HAS BEEN BIT BY A MAD DOG: Take a handful of the Herb call'd Ladies Bed-straw, bruise it in a Mortar; then roll up the Leaf and Juice, with a lump of butter, and make the Party swallow it. 'Tis sent to me as an immediate cure for Man or Beast.
A COLLECTION OF RECEIPTS IN COOKERY, PHYSICK AND SURGERY, LONDON 1749

Ladies Bedstraw is a common herb found in meadows and pastures in both Europe and North America. It is mentioned in Gerard's Herball (1597): 'There be divers sorts of herbs called Ladies Bedstraw or cheese renning.' It gets that second name because at one time in northern England, the flowers were used as a substitute for rennet to curdle milk in the making of cheese.

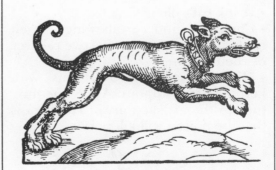

Rheumatism

Rheumatic diseases do abound
And through this distemper we see
  The Seasons alter

SHAKESPEARE, *A MIDSUMMER NIGHT'S DREAM*

Texans have a reputation for being big, strong and tough. When I consider many of their cures, like the ones that follow and others found throughout the book, I am convinced. They would have to be strong just to survive their own remedies.

TEXAS REMEDIES:
• Collect some pill bugs and fry them, then eat them.
• Take nine red peppers off stalks, one teaspoonful salt, one snuff box twiceful of coal oil and one teacup full of gasoline and mix and shake well. Rub this on where you hurt.
• Place a pan of chicken droppings under the bed.
• Bind joint with hot prickly pear poultice.
• Cut off the top of a toad stool and dry it. Wet it with whiskey and use it as a rub.
• Drink bat's blood.
• Chewing and swallowing dried rattlesnake flesh is an effective reliever of rheumatism.
• Mix a bucket of red ants with kerosene and sulphur. Apply the mixture to the afflicted area. The idea is that the poison will kill poison.

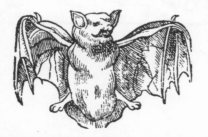

May seems to be the magic month for gathering ingredients. But, I would rather collect the May dew used in the freckle cures (pp.130-33) than the next ingredient.

TAKE COW DUNG gathered in May; put to it one third part of white wine and distil it. Give the patient four ounces going to rest. It is likewise good against the gout, stone and stoppage of the urine.
THE FAMILY MAGAZINE, LONDON 1741

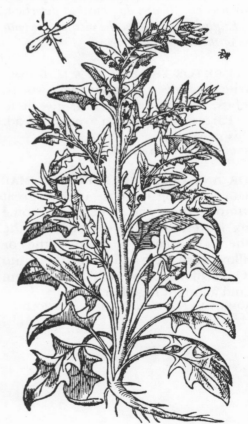

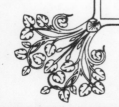
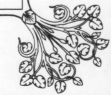

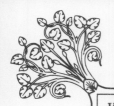

When the Europeans started exploring and colonizing the Americas and Australia, they brought tools, weapons and skills that were unknown to the native peoples. They also brought many strange new diseases, like smallpox, that wreaked havoc since the indigenous peoples had no natural resistance to them. But rheumatism was a malady common to all mankind, however the explanations and cures might vary. The Australian aborigines believed their rheumatic pains were caused by bits of stone or bone which some enemy had put in their footsteps. In North America, the native peoples taught the early white settlers their cures for rheumatism.

RED PEPPER POULTICE FOR RHEUMATISM: This remedy is supposed to have been learned from an old Indian squaw who had cured a case so bad the doctors had given it up. A large kettle is filled with water which is thickened to a poultice consistency with chopped red peppers and the mixture is boiled for an hour or so. Into this a linen sheet is dropped and placed steaming hot, about the body of the patient. In the meantime, blankets have been heated and with them a veritable inferno-bed prepared into which the patient is tightly tucked and fed cup after cup of hot tea until he sweats the rheumatism out of his system.
TENNESSEE REMEDY.

GREEN BAY INDIAN'S REMEDY: Wahoo, bark of the root, one ounce; blood root, one ounce; black cohosh root, two ounces; swamp hellebore, half an ounce, prickly ash, bark or berries, one ounce; poke root, cut fine, one ounce; rye whiskey, one quart; let stand a few days before using. Dose: one teaspoon every three to four hours, increasing the dose to two or three teaspoons as the stomach will bear.
DR CHASE'S RECIPES, 1867 EDITION

Dr. Chase incorrectly gave Euonymous Stropurpureous *as the botanical name for wahoo. This large shrub or small tree is actually* Euonymous Atropurpureus, *sometimes called burning bush. Hope that helps you find it.*

I also suspect that the rye whiskey was added to the original native cure. Several other cures for rheumatism include the white man's fire water. Perhaps it dulled the pain.

BITTERS FOR CHRONIC RHEUMATISM: Prickly-ash berries, spikenard root, yellow poplar and dog-wood barks, of each half a pound; all pulverized and put into a gallon jug and fill it with brandy. Dose: a wine glass of it is to be taken three times daily before meals.
DR CHASE'S RECIPES, 1867 EDITION

TAKE TWO HANDFULS OF ELECAMPANE, put it in three quarts of cider, boil it down to one quart. Take half a wineglassful three times a day. Very good.
A NUMBER OF RECEIPTS FOR CURING MAN AND BEAST, 1855.

In 1738, for some completely obscure reason, Jonathan Swift stated, 'kitchen physic is the best physic.' Potatoes and celery can certainly be found in most kitchens.

BATHE THE PARTS WITH WATER in which potatoes have been boiled, hot as can be borne, just before going to bed; by the morning the pain will be much relieved.
NEWSPAPER CLIPPING FROM A ONTARIO PIONEER'S SCRAPBOOK OF MEDICAL RECIPES, C. 1800

TRY A POTATO POULTICE for this painful disease. Boil two potatoes in their jackets. When done, mash potatoes—skins and all—spread on a cloth and apply.
LADIES HOME JOURNAL, PHILADELPHIA, MARCH 1890.

A POTATO CARRIED IN EACH POCKET till it turns to stone. It first becomes soft—afterwards as hard as a rock.
FROM A CANADIAN PIONEER'S DIARY.

A LADY IN NEW YORK writes that an eminent physician of her state has achieved quite a reputation for his success in treating cases of chronic rheumatism. His remedy is nothing more or less than the common celery. Boil some celery in water until it is quite soft and let the patient drink freely of the liquor three or four times a day. It is also beneficial when used as a food. Those suffering from rheumatism ought not to despair of a cure until they have tried this simple but effective remedy.
THE PEOPLE'S HOME MEDICAL BOOK, 1916

Liniments were rubbed directly on the affected areas.

LAMP OIL, SKUNK'S OIL AND RED PEPPER: For chronic rheumatism take two ounces of skunk's oil, the same quantity of cheap lamp oil and one teaspoonful of red pepper; shake well together and bathe with a piece of flannel dipped into this mixture.
THE PEOPLE'S HOME MEDICAL BOOK, 1916

TO MAKE RHEUMATIC LIQUID: One quart alcohol, one ounce spirit of turpentine, one ounce beef's gall, two ounces hartshorn, half an ounce camphor gum, half an ounce yellow cayenne pepper. To be put into a bottle and well shaken until all are dissolved. When used, rub it on parts affected two or three times a day. For the head-ache, bathe the top of the head with it.
DR. POWER'S IMPROVED MEDICINES, FOUND IN CANADIAN PIONEER DIARY, *C.* 1850

One cure still as popular today as it was in ancient times is bee stings. Rheumatism victims used to go directly to the bee keepers for treatment which, at least for the first dose, involved being stung twice.

One final word for those of you who are not afflicted with this painful condition. Never kick a cat or you will get rheumatism.

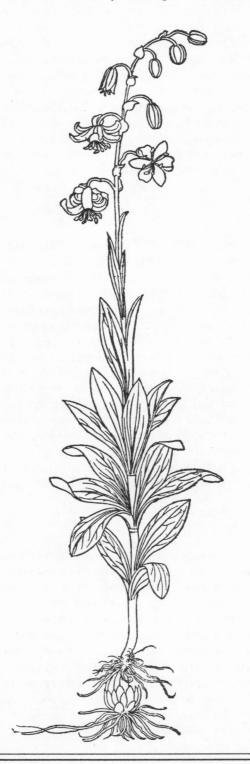

Ringworm

Ringworm has nothing to do with worms. Rather, it is a skin disease, caused by a fungus which does however grow in a circular or ring shape. When Dr Chase offered this first remedy to his readers, relations between the United States and Cuba were rather different. Americans now have to travel to Canada to buy the first ingredient.

TAKE THE BEST CUBA CIGARS, smoke one a sufficient length of time to accumulate ¼ to ½ inch of ash upon the end of the cigar; now wet the whole surface of the sore with saliva from the mouth then rub the ashes from the end of the cigar thoroughly into and all over the sore; do this three times a day, and inside of a week all will be smooth and well.
DR CHASE'S RECIPES, 1867 EDITION

Dr Chase added a warning. 'Tobacco is very valuable in its place (medicine), like spirits however, it makes slaves of its devotees.'

TEXAS REMEDIES:
• Take the saliva from a suckling calf and wash the infected area. Later wash with soap.
• Take a green walnut and cut a slice of it and rub it on the ringworm. Do this once or twice a day.
• Find a cat that died violently and rub the ringworms on the cat without moving it from its place.
• Rub the hot foam from fresh cow's milk on the spots.

WHISKEY, which has had Spanish-flies in soak, is said to be good for ringworm, but I've never known of an instance of it being tried. Unless too strong or used in great quantities, it cannot, at least do any harm. Washing the hands frequently in warm vinegar is good for ringworm.
LYDIA CHILD, *THE FRUGAL HOUSEWIFE*, BOSTON 1831

Lydia Child was a straightforward and honest woman who did not mince words. She dedicated her book "to Those Who Are not Ashamed of Economy" and included this verse.

Economy is a poor man's revenue,
extravagance a rich man's revenue.
And a word from the Reverend...

APPLY ROTTEN APPLES or pounded garlic.
OR, rub them with the juice of house-leek.
OR, wash them with Hungary water camphorated.
OR, twice a day with oil of sweet almonds and oil of tartar, mixed.
REVEREND JOHN WESLEY, PRIMITIVE PHYSICK, 1747

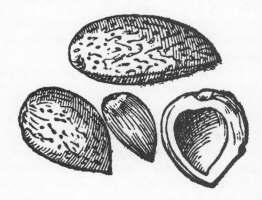

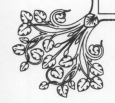
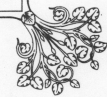

Sore Throat

'My sore throats, you know, are always worse than anybody's'
JANE AUSTEN (1775–1817), *PERSUASION*

A common complaint, sore throats are often treated by home remedies, including favourites such as a hot drink of honey and lemon or a gargle with salt water. An Australian standby is strong, hot tea as a gargle. However, if these old faithfuls bore you, perhaps you might find the following more inventive.

TAKE A SOCK you have worn into a boot and worked in for almost a week so that it has a bad odour. Tie it around your neck.
APPALACHIAN FOLK REMEDY

QUINSY OR SORE THROAT: Get three toads and tie them by the legs with a string. Let them stay in the sun until they decay away; wear the string around the neck. It is a simple and certain cure.
A NUMBER OF RECEIPTS FOR CURING MAN AND BEAST, 1855

TEXAS REMEDIES:
• Tie a black thread with nine knots in it around your neck. The thread should be dipped in turpentine.
• Have a complete stranger blow into the sick one's mouth.
• Tie a bag of red ants around the neck. After the ants are all dead, the throat will be well.
• Tie a string on a strip of bacon, swallow it and pull it back up.

The old proverb, 'Eat an apple going to bed, Make the doctor beg for his bread' has been modernized to 'An apple a day keeps the doctor away.' Apples, or pippins, as they were once called, were often recommended in sore throat cures.

A POWERFUL AND EXPERIENC'D MEDICINE FOR A SORE THROAT: Take two new-laid eggs roasted moderately hard, and the pap of two well roasted pippins: Beat them well together and add to them as much curds of posset made with ale. Having incorporated them all very well, apply the mixture very warm to the part affected, shifting it, if need be, once in five or six hours.
THE FAMILY MAGAZINE, LONDON, 1741

RECIPE FOR A PUTRID SORE THROAT: Mix one gill of strong apple cider, one tablespoonful of common salt, one tablespoonful of drained honey and half a pod of red pepper together boil them to a proper consistency, then pour it into half a pint of strong sage tea, take a teaspoonful occasionally and it will be found an infallible cure.
LADIES INDISPENSABLE ASSISTANT, NEW YORK, 1851

According to Reverend Wesley, an old sore throat could be cured by living wholly on apples and apple water. He also offered these alternatives.

TAKE A PINT of cold water lying down (Tried).
OR, apply a chin-stay of roasted figs.
OR, a flannel sprinkled with spirits of hartshorn to the throat, rubbing Hungary water on the top of the head.
OR, a flannel sprinkled with spirits of hartshorn to the throat, rubbing Hungary water on the top of the head.
OR, snuff a little honey up the nose.
REVEREND JOHN WESLEY, PRIMITIVE PHYSICK, 1747

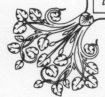

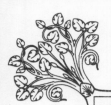

All of the following would certainly qualify as old grandmothers' cures, a commendation which Dr Chase warned us not belittle.

A GOOD OLD GRANDMOTHER'S GARGLE: Steep one medium sized red pepper in half a pint of water, strain and add ¼ pint of good vinegar, and a heaping teaspoonful each, of salt and pulverized alum, and gargle with it as often as needed.
DR CHASE'S RECIPES, 1892 EDITION

CUT SLICES OF SALT PORK or fat bacon; simmer a few moments in hot vinegar, and apply to throat as hot as possible. When this is taken off, as the throat is relieved, put around a bandage of soft flannel. A gargle of equal parts of borax and alum, dissolved in water, is also excellent. To be used frequently.
THE CANADIAN HOME COOK BOOK, 1877

MIX A QUARTER OF AN OUNCE OF SALT-PETRE, finely pulverized with three ounces of pure honey. Dilute it with vinegar and use it as a gargle: or take a small spoonful of it into the mouth occasionally and let it dissolve slowly.
FROM AN ONTARIO PIONEER'S SCRAPBOOK OF MEDICAL RECIPES

TAKE TWENTY DROPS of spirits of turpentine on loaf sugar every night until cured. Black currant jelly hastens the cure.
MERCHANT AND FARMERS ALMANACK, NEW BRUNSWICK, 1855

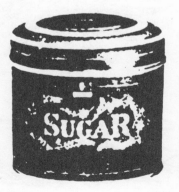

A sore throat often leads to hoarseness or even loss of voice; these remedies should take care of that.

LOSS OF VOICE: When the voice is lost, as is sometimes the case from the effects of cold, a simple pleasant remedy is furnished by beating up the white of one egg, adding to it the juice of one lemon, and sweetening it with white sugar to the taste. Take a teaspoonful from time to time.
THE FARMER'S ADVOCATE, LONDON, ONTARIO, AUGUST 1875

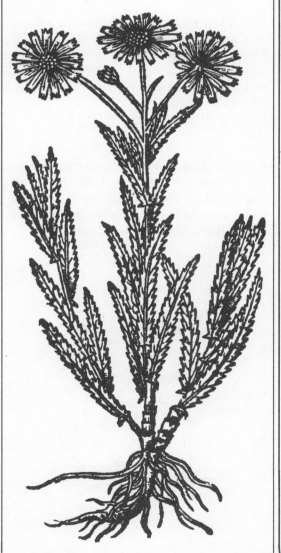

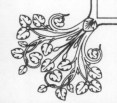

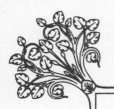

Stomach Troubles

(Also see Indigestion and Colic)

He who does not mind his belly will hardly mind anything else.
SAMUEL JOHNSON, *QUOTED BY BOSWELL*, 1763

TO CURE INFLAMMATION OF THE STOMACH: Drink the water in which onions have been boiled.
A NEW ENGLAND SIMPLE

FOR A SORE STOMACH: Take half a sheet of Cap-Paper, cut it in the Shape of a Heart, and dip it in Brandy and old candle grease melted together, of each an equal Quantity; apply it warm to the pit of the stomach.
THE COMPLETE FAMILY PIECE AND COUNTRY GENTLEMAN AND FARMER'S BEST GUIDE, LONDON 1741

FOR CRAMP IN THE STOMACH: Warm water sweetened with molasses or warm sugar, taken freely, will often remove the cramp in the stomach when opium and other medicines have failed.
THE LADY'S ANNUAL REGISTER, BOSTON 1838

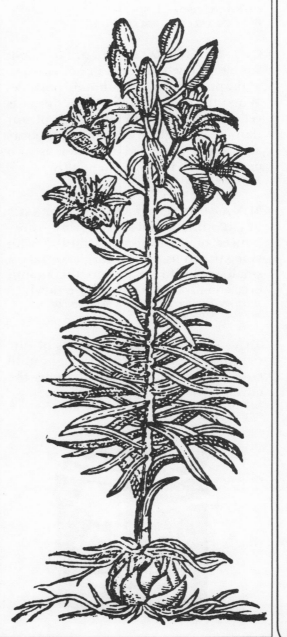

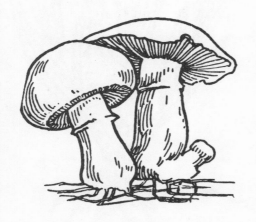

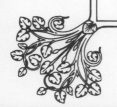

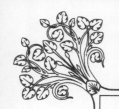

Toothache

For there was never yet philosopher
That could endure the toothache patiently
SHAKESPEARE, *MUCH ADO ABOUT NOTHING*

Toothache was simply a fact of life to our ancestors, at least until their teeth had all fallen out. After reading of the agonies our forefathers suffered with toothaches, we should all make more of an effort to smile, however weakly, at our dentists. This profession has the highest suicide rate, and quite possibly, the constant aura of rejection and distrust emanating from their patients is a contributing factor. Isn't a few minutes in the dentist's chair easier to contemplate than one of these remedies?

KENTUCKY REMEDIES:
• To cure toothache, cut a wart off a horse's leg and rub it on the gums.
• To cure toothache, choke a mole with your hands behind your head and hang one of its feet around your neck.
• If you stand a person against a tree and drive a nail into the tree just above his head, this process will cure toothache.
KENTUCKY SUPERSTITIONS, 1920

TO CURE THE TOOTHACHE, you must cut a little off each fingernail and toenail, and wrap it up in white paper and rise in the morning before sunrise, don't speak to any person or any person to you, and go towards sunrise and bore a hole in a thrifty oak tree and put the paper in the hole and drive a pin in the hole and use one of the highest names at each stroke, Father, Son and Holy Ghost.
JOHN STONER'S SYMPATHY, 1867

A GOOD REMEDY FOR THE TOOTHACHE: Stir the sore tooth with a needle until it draws blood; then take a thread and soak it with this blood. Then take vinegar and flour, mix them well so as to form a paste, and spread it on a rag, then wrap this rag around the root of an apple tree and tie it very close with the above thread, after which the root must be well covered with ground.
OR
Cut out a piece of greensvord (sod) in the morning before sunrise, quite unbeshrewedly from any place, breathe three times upon it and put it down upon the same place from which it was taken.
THE LONG LOST FRIEND, 1856

FOR TOOTHACHE AND NEURALGIA: Write down with a goose-quill and ink, new-made—but careful that nothing is wasted from the quill but what belongs to the shape of the pen—on the outside of the cheek, where the pain is situated, the following signs: mot, tot, fot. After this being done, light a candle, and precede therewith under the chimney. Burn the pen by the light under the hearth, until not a vestige thereof remains. All this must be done noiselessly, while the person who suffers the pain must at once put the head in a bandage, retire to bed, and remain quiet and by no means speak a word to anybody for twenty-four hours.
ALBERTUS MAGNUS OR EGYPTIAN SECRETS

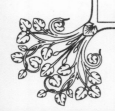
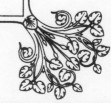

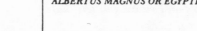

The man with the toothache thinks everyone happy whose teeth are sound.
SHAW, *MAXIMS FOR REVOLUTIONISTS*, 1903

AN INFALLIBLE CURE FOR TOOTH-ACHE: Wash the root of an aching tooth in elder vinegar and let it dry half an hour in the sun; after which it will never ache more.
BENJAMIN FRANKLIN, *POOR RICHARD'S ALMANACK*, PHILADELPHIA, 1739

One way to get rid of the problem is simply to get rid of the tooth. Until quite recently, a popular way of extracting a tooth was to attach a piece of string securely to the tooth with the other end tied to a doorknob. Slam the door, end of aching tooth. Here are some 'less painful' alternatives.

TO EXTRACT A TOOTH WITHOUT PAIN: Take some newts, by some called lizards, and those nasty beetles which are found in ferns in summertime. Calcine them in an iron pot and make a powder thereof. Wet the forefinger of the right hand and insert it in the powder and apply it to the tooth frequently, refraining from spitting it off, when the tooth will fall away without pain. It is proven.
OLD ENGLISH CURE

BURN A RED CORN COB to ashes and mix fresh lard with these ashes. Put this mixture on a piece of cotton and put it in the hollow of the tooth. This will stop the tooth from aching and will cure it by causing it to rot out.
TEXAS REMEDY

Incidentally, according to the Texans, if you trim your fingernails on Friday, you will not have a toothache for a week.

Getting rid of the terrible pain is the obsession of every sufferer. These promised blessed relief.

MAGNETIC TOOTH CORDIAL AND PAIN KILLER: Best alcohol, one ounce, laudanum $1/8$ ounce; gum camphor, half an ounce, oil of cloves, half a dram; sulphuric ether, $3/4$ ounce; and oil of lavender, one dram. If there is a nerve exposed, this will quiet it. Apply with lint. Rub also on the gums and upon the face against the tooth, freely.
DR CHASE'S RECIPES, 1867 EDITION

Plain oil of cloves is still used to help numb the teeth until the dentist can squeeze us in. While you wait, practice this rhyme that Dr Chase added at the end of his cure.
The raging toothache why now endure
 when there is found a perfect cure,
Which saves the tooth and stops the
 pain,
 and gives the sufferer ease again.

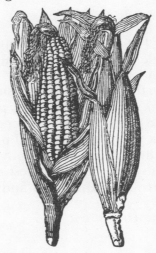

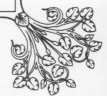

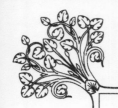

Who hath aching teeth hath ill tenants.
ENGLISH PROVERB

FIELDTHISTLE: The worst case of toothache can be cured by chewing a piece of the root of a large field thistle which is commonly known as 'bull thistle'; and by drinking a tea and applying a poultice made from its leaves you can permanently cure the worst case of neuralgia that ever existed. Give it a trial and be convinced.
THE PEOPLE'S HOME MEDICAL BOOK, CLEVELAND, 1916

SPLIT A RAISON, put a little mustard on the sticky side and apply to the aching tooth or gum. It will draw out all the soreness: or; boil either a raison or a small fig in milk and apply to the tooth while hot.
THE PEOPLE'S HOME MEDICAL BOOK, CLEVELAND, 1916

INFALLIBLE CURE FOR THE TOOTHACHE: One-quarter pound pale peruvian bark finely powdered; one pint of old 4th proof French brandy, one pint of rosewater; one pint of pure water. Mix and after twenty-four hours, it is fit for use. For severe toothache, add one to four more brandy in proportion to any given quantity of the above, which hold in mouth five minutes.
THE CANADIAN FARMER'S ALMANAC, 1825

RINSE YOUR MOUTH with your own urine three mornings and the teeth will never again ache. The above will not cure decayed teeth.
Fill a pipe half full of tobacco, then put a little brimstone into it and the pipe up with tobacco, light it and hold the smoke in the mouth as long as possible.
MRS (REVEREND) B. SMITH, NEWFOUNDLAND, 1841

Even before we get our teeth, they're causing us grief.

A GOOD WAY TO CAUSE CHILDREN TO CUT THEIR TEETH WITHOUT PAIN: Boil the brain of a rabbit and rub the gums of the children with it, and their teeth will grow without pain to them.
THE LONG LOST FRIEND, 1856

CUTTING TEETH: Make a necklace of the bean called Job's Tears and let the child wear it around it's neck.
LADIES INDISPENSABLE ASSISTANT, NEW YORK, 1852

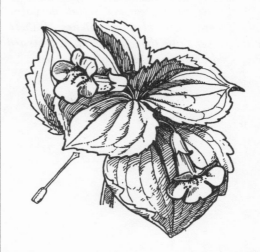

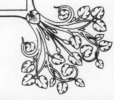

TO MAKE NECKLACES FOR CHILDREN IN CUTTING TEETH: Take roots of henbane, orpin, and vervain; scrape them clean with a sharp knife, cut them in long beads, and string them green; first henbane, then orpin, then vervain, and so do 'till 'tis the bigness of the child's neck. Then take as much red wine as you think the necklace will suck up, and put into it a dram of red coral, as much single peony root finely powder'd soak your beads in this twenty-eight hours and rub the powder on the beads. Syrup of lemons and syrup of single peony are excellent to rub the child's gums with very frequently.

THE COMPLETE FAMILY PIECE AND COUNTRY GENTLEMAN AND FARMER'S BEST GUIDE, LONDON, 1741

Henbane, orpine and vervain were supposed to have many magical powers. Henbane was also popular in treating adult toothache, because it was believed that the pain was caused by tiny worms which the henbane expelled. Orpine was often called Live-Long because it remains green for quite a while after being cut. It was an English custom to gather it on Midsummer's Eve and hang it up in the house as protection against disease and also lightning. Vervain was known as a holy plant after the Crusaders brought back the story that vervain sprang up on Calvary when the nails were driven into Christ's hands. It was believed to ward off the evil eye as indicated in this verse: 'Trefoil, vervain, John's wort, dill, Hinder witches of their will.' 'Not so,' said the witches. They, it turned out, used vervain, in most of their brews.

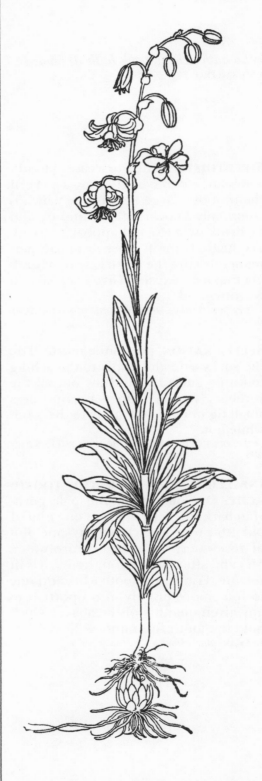

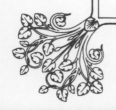

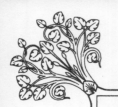

Vomiting

One ov the best temporary cures for pride and affectashun that i hav ever seen tried is sea-sickness; a man who wants tew vomit, never puts on airs.
JOSH BILLINGS, *ODS AND ENS* (1818-85)

Remedies for vomiting fall into two distinct categories. The cure is either applied externally to the stomach or a potion is swallowed. Some of the old remedy books suggest both treatments at the same time, perhaps from the knowledge that it is very difficult to convince someone with an upset stomach to swallow anything.

APPLY A LARGE ONION, slit, to the pit of the stomach. Or. Use a Spoonful of Juice of Lemon, and six grains of salt of wormwood.
THE HOUSEKEEPER'S POCKET BOOK—EVERYONE THEIR OWN PHYSICIAN, C. 1750

POUND UP GUM CAMPHOR, pour on boiling water; sweeten it with loaf sugar, and let the patient take a spoonful every ten minutes. A drink made of common pigweed is said to be a good remedy; also a mustard poultice applied to the pit of the stomach, is good.
BROCKVILLE ALMANAC, 1867

Mustard poultices or plasters are more often used for colds and chest congestion. To make a mustard plaster, mix equal parts of ground mustard and flour into a paste with warm water and spread between two pieces of cloth, preferably flannel or muslin.

TAKE A LARGE NUTMEG, grate away half of it and then toast the flat side till the Oil ouze out; then clap it to the Pit of the Stomach. Let it lie so long as 'tis warm, repeat it often until cured.
THE COMPLETE FAMILY PIECE AND COUNTRY GENTLEMAN AND FARMER'S BEST GUIDE, LONDON, 1741

Incidentally, according to English folklore, changes in the dreamer's life are foretold by dreams of nutmeg.

FOR VOMITING AND DIARRHEA: Take pulverized cloves and eat them together with bread soaked in red wine, and you will soon find relief. The cloves may be put on bread.
THE LONG LOST FRIEND, 1856

A well-known Australian cure is to swallow neat a tablespoon of burnt brandy. The Australian Country Women's Association Cook Book advises: 'To burn brandy, put about one and a half tablespoons of brandy in a saucer and set it alight. When the flame dies, the brandy is ready for use.'

Brandy is also included in this remedy for seasickness. And who knows, today, it may work for airsickness also.

TO PREVENT SEA-SICKNESS: Make a pad of wool or horse hair and bind it over the stomach. Brandy and water very weak is the best remedy to allay the heat and irration.
BUCKEYE COOKERY, MINNEAPOLIS, 1881

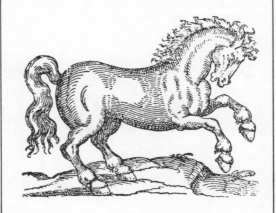

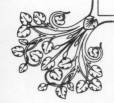
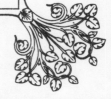

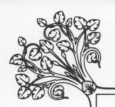
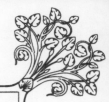

Warts

One who expects his friends not to be offended by his own warts, will pardon the other's pimples.
HORACE, 35 BC

There are enough superstitions and cures for warts to fill a whole book alone. Why would warts attract such an extensive collection of folklore? Perhaps because of their inexplicable appearance and disappearance. Modern medicine has discovered that warts are caused by a viral infection of the skin. They quite often disappear spontaneously, so it is quite understandable that if the cure coincides with the natural disappearance, the remedy will be given the credit.

A GOOD OINTMENT FOR SERIOUS WARTS: Make a white turnip hollow inside by taking the pit out, put fresh butter therein, also a fresh hen's egg. Let these articles be rendered by broiling inside, pour through a cloth, with a little rose water added, and boil it till it becomes the consistency of a salve. This is a very reliable ointment.
ALBERTUS MAGNUS OR EGYPTIAN SECRETS

A SIMPLE CURE FOR WARTS: Cut a piece of wild turnip, from the woods, and rub several times upon the wart or warts.
DR CHASE'S RECIPES, 1892 EDITION

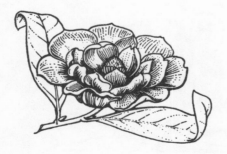

These folk remedies come from Redwood Country, California.

• Put a dead cat under a porch during a full moon and it will remove warts from your hand.
• Cut your wart in half and bury one half of it at a fork in the road at midnight. The buried half of the wart will keep sucking blood out of the other half, and the wart will die.
• To get rid of a wart, tie a knot around the wart and say a prayer in the Bible. The wart will disappear within three days.

IF YOU RUB WARTS with fig-leaves and bury the said leaves in the earth, the warts will go away as the leaves rot.
THE HOUSEKEEPER'S ALMANAC, NEW YORK, 1842

DISSOLVE AS MUCH COMMON WASHING SODA as the water will take up. Wash the hands or warts with this for a minute or two, and allow them to dry without being wiped. This is repeated twice a day for a few days in succession, will gradually, but certainly destroy the most irratable warts.
MERCHANT AND FARMER'S ALMANACK, NEW BRUNSWICK, 1855

WASH THE HANDS in the moon's rays focussed in a dry metal basin saying.
I wash my hands in this thy dish,
O Man in the moon do grant my wish,
And come and take away this
ENGLISH CHARM CURE FROM CORNWALL

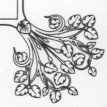

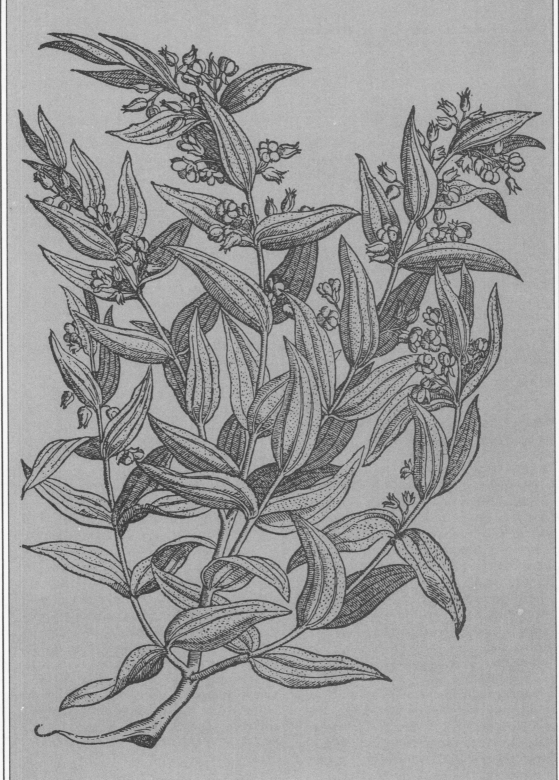

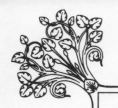

"Alas, poor chin! many a wart is richer.'
SHAKESPEARE, *TROILUS AND CRESSIDA*

TINCTURE OF CANTHARIDES, with some drops of tincture of iodine; apply to warts with a small brush or a little stick three or four times a day. In a few days, the warts will disappear.
THE HEARTHSTONE, PHILADELPHIA, 1883

RUB THEM DAILY with a radish, or with the juice of marigold flowers—it will hardly fail. Or, water in which sal-ammoniac is dissolved. Or, apply bruised purslain as a poultice, changing it twice a day. It cures in seven or eight days.
DR CHASE'S RECIPES, 1880 EDITION.

Dr Chase gave credit to Reverend John Wesley for these remedies. Sometimes he didn't bother to tell his readers that his cures were not original.

TEXAS REMEDIES:
• Go into a cornfield on a clear night under a full moon and catch a frog. Kill it, cut off its hind legs and save it until the next full moon. Then go out again, catch a cricket, and kill it and cut off its right hind leg. Put both legs under your pillow. Wake every hour and change their positions. After doing this for twelve hours, sleep for six more hours and the warts will be gone upon awakening.
• The only way to get rid of warts is to sell them.
• Rub grasshopper spit on a wart twice a day and it will leave in two weeks.
• Take a tick from a dog and let the tick bite the wart. Two or three days later the wart should have vanished. You then put the tick back on the dog.

• Rub the wart with an apple. Store the apple in the attic and when the apple is rotten, the wart will be gone.

There was an old English belief that warts were indicators of good or bad luck according to their position on the body. A wart on the right hand meant riches were to be expected. One on the face was believed to denote troubles of various kinds—as if the embarrassment of a wart on your nose were not trouble enough!

MULLEIN: The juice of the leaves and flowers being laid upon rough warts, also the powder of the dried roots rubbed on, doth easily take them away, but doth no good to smooth warts. Garden Rue: Taketh away all sorts of warts if boiled in wine with some pepper and nitre and the place rubbed therewil and with almond and honey.
NICHOLAS CULPEPER, *THE ENGLISH PHYSICIAN,* 1652

MILKWEED: Bruise milkweed and apply the milk that runs from them to the warts several times a day and they will soon come off. Ashes and vinegar: Burn some common willow bark, mix the ashes with a strong vinegar and apply frequently. Cinnamon Oil: Apply it several times a day for a week or more. A lady living in Garrettsville, Ohio, says she cured a seed wart with this. It must be used some time, but will effect a cure. Rosinweeds: The milk from rosin weeds frequently applied will remove warts.
THE PEOPLE'S HOME MEDICAL BOOK, CLEVELAND 1916

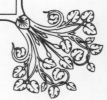

For since he would sit on a prophet's seat,
As a lord of the human soul,
We needs must scan him from head to feet,
Were it but for a wart or mole.
TENNYSON, *THE DEAD PROPHET*

TO CURE WARTS, take half an ounce of sulphur, half an ounce of 90% spirits. Put into an ounce phial, shake them well together, and then freely apply to the affected parts or warts for a few days once or twice a day and in a few weeks or months at most, the wart will disappear.
FROM CANADIAN PIONEER DIARY

A notation beside this diary entry said that the remedy had been copied from the 23 August 1853 issue of the New York Tribune.

GO INTO A FIELD and take a black snail, and rub them with the same nine times one way, and then nine times another and then stick that said snail upon a black thorn and the warts will waste. I have also known a black snail cure corns, being laid thereon as a plaister. If you have what is called blood or bleeding warts, then take a piece of raw beef that never had any salt, and rub them with the same just in the same manner as you used the snail above mentioned; after this operation is performed, you must bury that piece of beef in the earth.
THE FAMILY PHYSICIAN, 1814

After picking each wart with a pin, stick the pins into the bark of an ashen tree and repeat this old English charm cure:

Ashen tree, ashen tree,
Pray buy these warts of me

KENTUCKY FOLK REMEDIES:
• Rub the warts with a piece of bacon. Tie a string around the bacon and bury it secretly. The warts will leave within nine days.
• To cure warts, rub seven grains of corn on the warts, then feed the corn to your neighbour's chickens.
• If you have warts, wait until someone dies; then just at midnight, go to the graveyard and call to the devil. He will take away the warts.
• If you kiss your wart and then kiss someone, your wart will come off.
• Throw a piece of potato over your left shoulder. When the potato sprouts, your wart will be cured.
• To cure a wart, walk backwards in the moonlight to an old stump full of water and stick your hand into the stump.

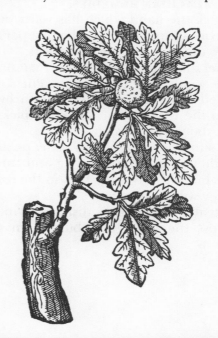

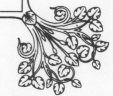

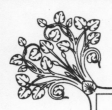
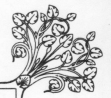

Remark all these roughnesses, pimples, warts, and everything as you see me, otherwise I will never pay a farthing for it.
OLIVER CROMWELL'S INSTRUCTION TO PAINTER SIR PETER LELY

RECEIPT TO CURE WARTS: Take the inner rind of a lemon, steep it for four and twenty hours in distilled vinegar, and apply it to the warts. It must not be left on the part above three hours at a time, and it is to be applied fresh every day. Or divide a red onion, and rub the warts with it, or anoint them with the milky juice of the herb mercury several times and they will gradually waste away.
THE FAMILY PHYSICIAN AND FARMER'S COMPANION,
SYRACUSE, NEW YORK, C. 1840

TO DESTROY WARTS: Roast chicken feet and rub the warts with them, then bury them under the eaves.
THE LONG LOST FRIEND, 1856

APPALACHIAN REMEDIES:
• Stick the hand which has warts on it into a bag and tie it up. The first person who opens it will get your warts.
• Get something like a penny that someone would like to pick up. Put some blood from the wart on it and throw it into the road. When someone picks it up, the wart will go away.
• Count the warts. Tie as many pebbles as there are warts in a bag and throw this bundle down in a fork in the road. They will soon go away.
• Steal a neighbour's dishrag. Wipe it across the warts and bury it in the woods.

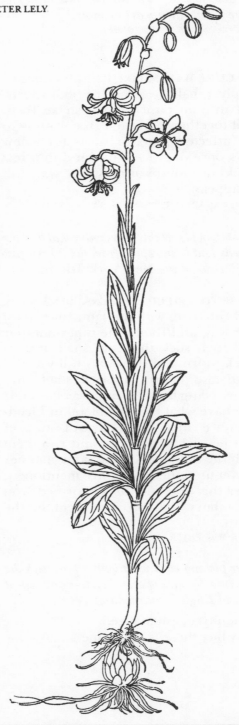

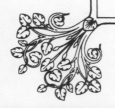

Whooping Cough

Whooping cough is a childhood disease also known as chin-cough or pertussis. For some strange reason, it is more common in girls. An infectious disease of the mucus membrane lining the air passage, whooping cough got that name from the peculiar convulsive cough and loud indrawing of breath of its small victims.

In his History of Medicine, *William Black (1771-1811) said; 'up to this century the management of these tender creatures in sickness was left to ignorant old nurses and rude quackery.' These cures for whooping cough would probably fall within Mr Black's definition.*

LET THE PARENT OF THE AFFLICTED CHILD catch a spider and hold it over the head of the child, repeating three times.

'Spider as you waste away,
whooping cough no longer stay.'
The spider must then be hung up in a bag over the mantlepiece and when it has dried up, the cough will have disappeared.
OLD ENGLISH REMEDY

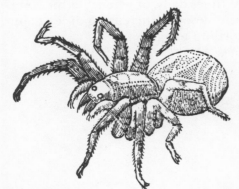

TO BANISH THE WHOOPING COUGH: Cut three small bunches of hair from the crown of the head of the child that has never seen its father; sew this hair up in an unbleached rag and hang it around the neck of the child having the whooping cough. The thread with which the rag is sewed must also be unbleached.

ANOTHER REMEDY FOR THE WHOOPING COUGH: Which has cured the majority of those who have applied it. Thrust the child having the whooping cough three times through a blackberry bush without speaking or saying anything. The bush, however, must be grown fast at the two ends, and the child must be thrust through three times in the same manner, that is to say, from the same side it was thrust through in the first place.
THE LONG LOST FRIEND, 1856

TO KEEP OFF WHOOPING COUGH, wear a black velvet band around the neck. Or, a tea made from white ants will cure whooping cough.
KENTUCKY SUPERSTITIONS, 1920

This next cure was sent to me by Mrs M. Sharp of New South Wales, Australia, who said she was saved from whooping cough at the age of six months by this old Scottish Wive's Tale.

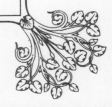

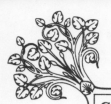

GO OUT INTO THE WET FOREST WILD PLACES and collect wild garlic. Dig it out to the white little bulbs. Cut both white and fresh green stalks up small—¼ inch—bits and put small heap on two pads of gauze so as to make two small poultices. Bind these while fresh and juicy to the soles of the child's feet, then put old cotton socks over to keep them on. Change to fresh poultices once every day.

Mrs. Sharp added, 'Some children get over the worst in twelve hours, others take three days, but they stink terribly of garlic.'
While not as dramatic, these syrups and potions sound more reasonable for easing convulsive coughing.

A TEASPOONFUL OF CASTOR OIL to a tablespoon of molasses, a teaspoon of the mixture to be given whenever the cough is troublesome. It will afford relief at once and in a few days it effects a cure. The same remedy relieves the croup, however violent the attack.
THE CANADA FARMER, TORONTO, 19 JUNE 1847

THE BEST KIND OF COFFEE prepared as for the table and given as a common drink to the child as warm as it can be drunk; and a piece of alum, for the patient to lick as often as it may wish. Most children are fond of alum, and will get all they need without being urged, but if they dislike it, they must be made to taste of it eight or ten times in the course of the day. It will effectually break up the worst case of whooping cough in a very short time.
AVERY'S ALMANACK FOR 1857, SAINT JOHN, NEW BRUNSWICK.

The Almanack added this caution: 'To adults or children in the habit of taking coffee, the remedy is good for nothing.'

CHESTNUT LEAVES, one ounce, water, one quart. Let it come to a boil and set aside in a teapot. Drink freely, hot or cold, the more the better and at all times day and night. It is said to effectually cure the disease in two weeks.
NEWSPAPER CLIPPING IN CANADIAN PIONEER'S DIARY

Settlers learned of the virtues of chestnut tea from the Indian, who also used it as both a tonic and sedative.

WHOOPING COUGH SYRUP: Make a syrup of prickly pear and drink freely. Take about three moderate sized leaves of the prickly pear to a quart of cold water, cut up in pieces and boil slowly about half an hour, strain out all the prickles thru' close muslin or linen, sweeten with white sugar and boil, a little longer. A safe and sure cure, and so pleasant to taste, that infants will take it with relish.
DR CHASE'S RECIPES, 1892 EDITION.
OR
ONIONS AND GARLIC, sliced of each, one gill; sweet oil, one gill; stew them in the oil in a covered dish to obtain the juices, then strain and add honey, one gill; paregoric and spirits of camphor, of each half an ounce; bottle and cork tight for use. Dose: for children of two to three years, one teaspoon three or four times daily, or whenever the cough is troublesome, increasing or lessening, according to age.
DR CHASE'S RECIPES, 1867 EDITION

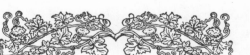

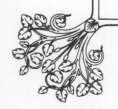

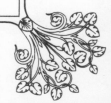

Today parents are advised to let children breathe the steam from a hot shower turned full force. A trip to the bathroom is certainly easier, and probably safer, than this last cure.

A REMARKABLE CURE: It is said that physicians in Paris have discovered a certain specific for whooping cough. The child is sent to a neighbouring gas manufactory to inhale for a few minutes the vapours which arise for the lime used to purify gas. Two or three visits effect a radical cure.
FROM A SCRAPBOOK OF MEDICAL RECIPES

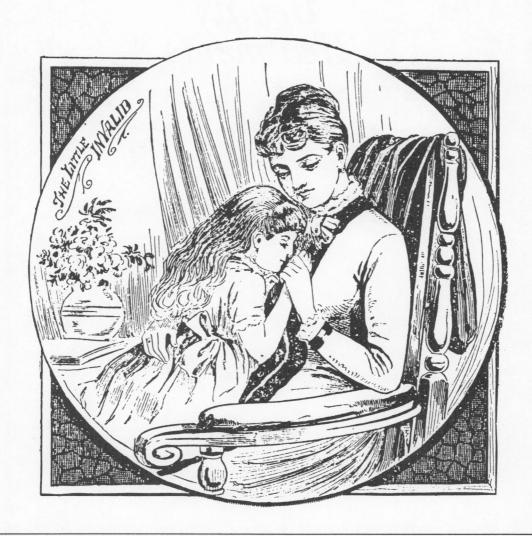

THE LITTLE INVALID.

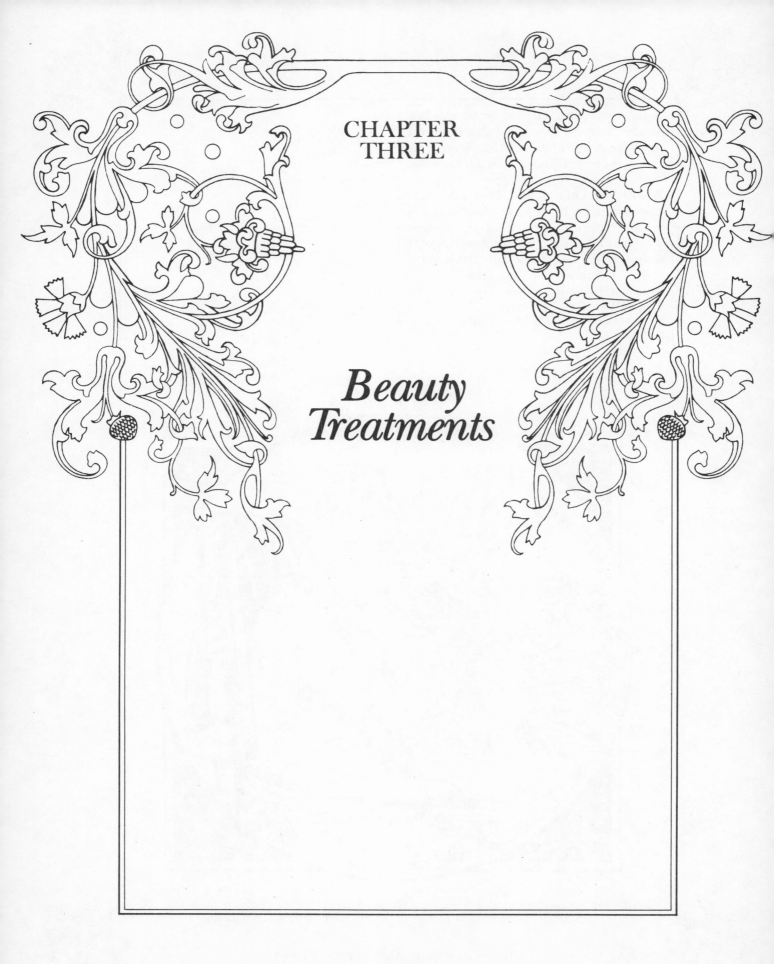

CHAPTER
THREE

*Beauty
Treatments*

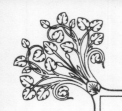

Call it vanity, narcissim or conceit, but most people are conscious of their appearance, even if not concerned about it. We suffer most acutely from this self-awareness during adolescence, but doubts about our looks never leave us. And we are probably more likely to experiment with potions and lotions which alter our looks than with medicinal brews. Who hasn't tried a little beer on the hair to give it more bounce and lustre, a face pack concocted of eggs or avocados, a little lemon juice on the hair to get that California sun-bleached look, or been willing to try almost anything to get rid of pimples? And although worship of the youthful image has reached levels of total absurdity today, even Horace was fretting about wrinkles in 23 BC.

In this section we find remedies for pimples, freckles, baldness, wrinkles, chapped lips, bruised nails, bad breath and loose teeth using ingredients which range from the delightful—May dew, rose petals and strawberries—to the thoroughly unpleasant—cow manure and urine! Things have a way of coming full circle. After years of promoting an endless number of expensive commercial products containing exotic synthetic chemicals, suddenly manufacturers of beauty products boast of the 'natural ingredients' in their latest preparations. Old-grandmother recipes triumph once more.

I dedicate this section to Kin Hubbard, who said: 'Beauty is only skin deep, but it's a valuable asset if you're poor and haven't any sense.'

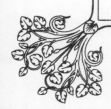
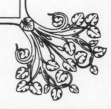

Face

COMPLEXION

Contentment is the best powder for a woman's face
DUTCH PROVERB

In these days of air pollution, food additives, central heating and its drying effects, plus the stresses of 20th century living, it sometimes takes more than contentment to enhance the complexion. But the large number of home remedies I have found for complexion, blemishes and wrinkles suggests that we have always been discontented with our skin and have tried to improve on nature. However, as Dr Chase suggests, simply being in tune with nature will do a lot to improve your complexion.

BE CHEERFUL; get as much fresh air in-doors and out-doors as possible. Keep in health; promote a good digestion and regular evacuations, avoid alcoholic drinks; a milk and vegetable diet makes a fair complexion; plain living without condiments and hot seasoning etc make the fairest face. It is good to rise early, drink a cup of milk, walk into the fields, wash the face in sparkling dew, gaze on creation below, above and all around you until mental pleasure beams forth on your face in radiant smiles. Check the effects of grief, disappointments, embarrassments etc.
DR CHASE'S RECIPES, 1880 EDITION

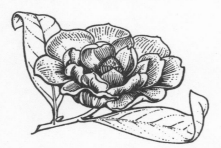

Throughout history, fashion has been fickle. What once was thought ugly, suddenly becomes fashionable. Today, a beautiful dark tan is a status symbol associated with luxurious winter vacations or summer weekends on the yacht. At one time, ladies avoided the coarsening effects of the sun at all costs. And if they were unlucky enough to have a swarthy complexion, they would possibly have resorted to one of the following.

AN EXCELLENT RECIPE TO CLEAR A TANNED SKIN: At night, going to bed, bathe the face with the juice of strawberries and let it lie on the part all night, and in the morning wash yourself with Chervil Water. The skin will soon become fair and smooth.
OLD PAMPHLET ON COSMETICS

This is a good treatment to remember because both strawberries and the herb chervil are also believed to combat wrinkles.

TO MAKE A SWARTHY COMPLEXION APPEAR AGREEABLE: Sift the flour out of half a peck of wheatbran, then put to the bran eight new laid eggs, and six pints of white wine vinegar, let the eggs be beaten as small as possible, and when the whole is properly mixed, let it distil over a slow fire, when it has stood a day to settle, take a little of it and rub your face every day for a fortnight and it will look extremely fair.
THE COMPLEAT VERMIN KILLER AND USEFUL POCKET COMPANION, DUBLIN, 1778

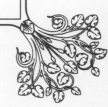

Cold water, morning and evening, is the best of all cosmetics
HEBREW PROVERB

A WASH FOR LADIES TO OBTAIN A FAIR AND BEAUTIFUL PHYSIOGONOMY: Take bread crumbs, put them into goat's milk whey, strain or distil it, paint the face with it, and it will become fair and beautiful.
ALBERTUS MAGNUS OR EGYPTIAN SECRETS

THE FIRST OR ORDINARY LUPINE do the scoure and cleanse the skin from spots, morphew, blew markes and other discolouring thereof, being used either in decoction or powder. We seldome use it in inward medicines, not that it is dangerous, but of neglect, for formerly it hathe been much used.
JOHN PARKINSON, *THE GARDEN OF PLEASANT FLOWERS*, 1629

BEAUTY RECIPE TO CLEAR THE SKIN: Half a pound of pumpkin pealing, two midleing carrots boiled in two quarts water until done. Put into a pitcher three rusty spikes and three rusty nails, put the pot liquor of the above on the spikes and nails. Give a wineglass full four times a day.
OLD MEDICAL RECIPE FROM RHODE ISLAND, 1831

A GOOD THING TO WASH THE FACE IN: Take a large piece of camphire, the quantity of a Goose Egg, and break it so that it may go into a Pint Bottle, which fill with water. When it has stood a Month, put a spoonful of it in three spoonfuls of milk and wash with it. Wear a piece of lead, beaten exceedingly thin, for a Fore-head Piece, under the Fore-head Cloth, it keeps the Fore-head smooth and plump.
THE COMPLETE FAMILY PIECE AND COUNTRY GENTLEMAN AND FARMER'S BEST GUIDE, LONDON, 1741

A COSMETIC JUICE: Make a hole in a lemon, fill it with Sugar Candy and close it nicely with leaf gold applied over the rind that was cut out; then roast the Lemon in hot ashes. When desirous of using the juice, squeeze out a little through the hole and wash the face with a napkin wetted with it. This juice greatly cleanses the skin and brightens the complexion.
OLD PAMPHLET ON COSMETICS

Considering the price of gold these days, perhaps a piece of aluminum foil could be substituted for the leaf gold. As you will see later, lemon juice was also a popular freckle cure.

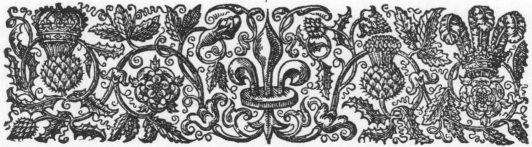

It wasn't enough to have fair complexion. It also had to be translucent, shiny and radiant. And here are some of the ways the ladies achieved that look.

TO MAKE POMATUM TO BEAUTIFY THE FACE: Take a handful of oats, and stick them in the fat of a bacon hog, newly killed, without any salt, let it melt before a slow fire and when it is quite dissolved, put to the drippings a spoonful of the oil of cinnamon, with the same quantity of the oil of sweet almonds, when you have mixed all these together, let it be laid up and it will make a most excellent pomatum.
THE COMPLEAT VERMIN KILLER AND USEFUL POCKET COMPANION, DUBLIN, 1778

The reader should note that animal fat, especially lard, may stimulate the growth of superfluous hair.

A COSMETIK WONDERFUL TO MAKE A PLEASING RUDDY COMPLEXION: Take madder, Myrrh, Saffron, Frankincense, of each alike, bruise or steep all in White-wine, with which anoint the face going to bed and in the morning, wash it off, and the skin will have a gallant pleasing blush.
POLYGRAPHICES, WILLIAM SALMON

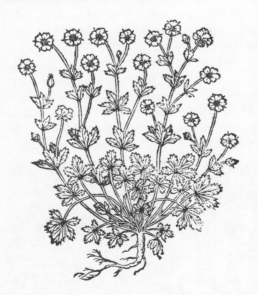

AN ADMIRABLE VARNISH FOR THE SKIN: Take equal parts of Lemon juice and whites of new laid eggs, beat them well together in a glased earthen pan, which put on a slow fire, and keep the mixture constantly stirring with a wooden spatula, till it has acquired the consistence of soft butter. Keep it for use and at the time of applying it, add a few drops of any essence you like best. Before the face be rubbed with this varnish, it will be proper to wash with the distilled water of rice. This is one of the best methods of rendering the complexion fair and the skin smooth, soft and shining.
OLD PAMPHLET ON COSMETICS, FOUND IN ONTARIO ARCHIVES

Beautiful complexion shouldn't stop at the neck! White flawless skin should continue right down to the toes. And it is best to start the treatment while young, as the following recipe suggests.

SKINNE KEPT WHITE AND CLEAR: Wash the face and body of a suckling child with brest milke or cowe milke, or mixed with water, every night, and the childe's skinne will waxe faire and cleare, and resist sunburning.
SIR HUGH PLATT, DELIGHTS FOR LADIES, 1609

TO MAKE THE SHOULDERS AND BREASTS APPEAR WHITE: Take a quart of dew gathered in May, with half a pint of fumitory water, put to them two ounces of lavender-water, then let all the ingredients be properly mixed and put up in a vessel to settle. Wash your neck, breast and shoulders first in the water that chammomile flowers have been boiled in, mixed with white wine, let it dry in and then rub this liquid upon it and the skin will appear quite transparent.
THE COMPLEAT VERMIN KILLER AND USEFUL POCKET GUIDE, DUBLIN, 1778

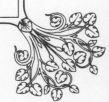

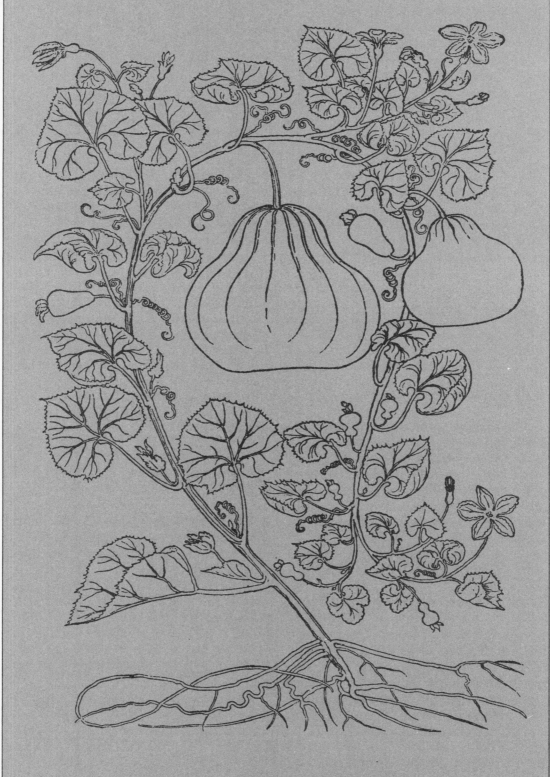

PIMPLES

Even the fairest of complexions are marred if spotted with pimples. According to Dr Chase, 'They generally arise from indigestion, or some internal derangement; therefore the disease should be attacked at the root. He suggested the following remedy.

TINCTURE OF CARDOMONS, one drachm; ipecacuanha wine and a teaspoonful of flour of sulphur, with a glass of sherry or ginger wine. Take this on going to bed; repeat it every second or third night, and keep the bowels gently open.
DR CHASE'S RECIPES, 1880 EDITION.

Cardomom is a perennial herb, native to southern India and used mainly as an ingredient in curry powder. Ipecacuanha is a plant indigenous to Brazil and its name is taken from the native word meaning 'roadside sick-making plant'. It was a popular cure for dysentery.

Most pimple preparations were to be applied directly on the offending spots, as in these cures.

HOW TO TAKE AWAY LITTLE RED SPOTS FROM THE FACE: Take two ounces of lemon juice, two ounces of rose water, two drachms of silver suppliment, mix them into an ointment and rub your face with the same on going to bed, and when you get up in the morning rub your face with fresh butter, and then rub the same clean off.
DR. PARKINS, *THE FAMILY PHYSICIAN,* 1814

AN OINTMENT WHICH IS A CERTAIN CURE FOR ANY SCABS, PIMPLES OR OLD INVETERATE ITCH: Take a quarter of an Ounce of Red Precipitate, grind it on a Marble Stone, till 'tis as fine as the flour of brimstone and work up both with three ounces of Butter without salt, as it comes from the Churn; mix it very well, and Anoint the place very thin with the Ointment. Tis not the Nature of it to check, but draw out the Distemper; and in a Week or Ten Days Confinement, will make an absolute cure. I should say many things to Recommend this, being sure of its virtues, but it will not need that, to any body of Judgement.
MRS MARY KETTIBY, *A COLLECTION OF RECEIPTS IN COOKERY, PHYSICK AND SURGERY,* LONDON, 1749

Red Precipitate is mercuric oxide or red oxide of mercury.

A REMEDY FOR PIMPLES: Take half a quarter of a Pound of Bitter Almonds, blanch, stamp them, and put them into half a pint of Spring-water, stir it together, and strain it out; then put to it half a pint of the best Brandy, and a pennyworth of the Flour of Brimstone. Shake it well when you use, which must be often. Dab it on with a fine rag.
THE COMPLETE FAMILY PIECE AND COUNTRY GENTLEMAN AND FARMER'S BEST GUIDE, LONDON, 1741

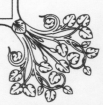

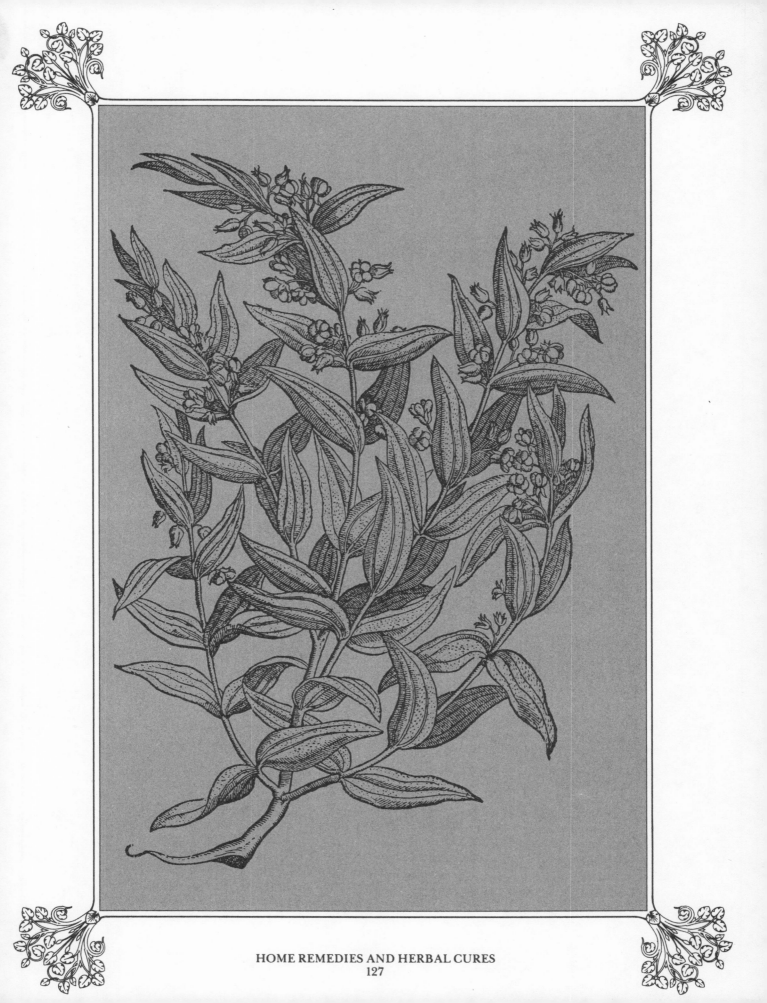

A WATER FOR PIMPLES IN THE FACE:
Boil together a handful of the herbs
Patience and Pimpernel in water; and
wash yourself every day with the decoc-
tion.
OLD PAMPHLET OF COSMETIC RECIPES, ONTARIO
ARCHIVES

*Pimpernel, an herb, is better known as great
burnet and is used mainly as an astringent
and tonic.*

CUT A BEAN IN HALF; place half of it on
the pimple and bury the other half. The
pimple will be gone in the morning.

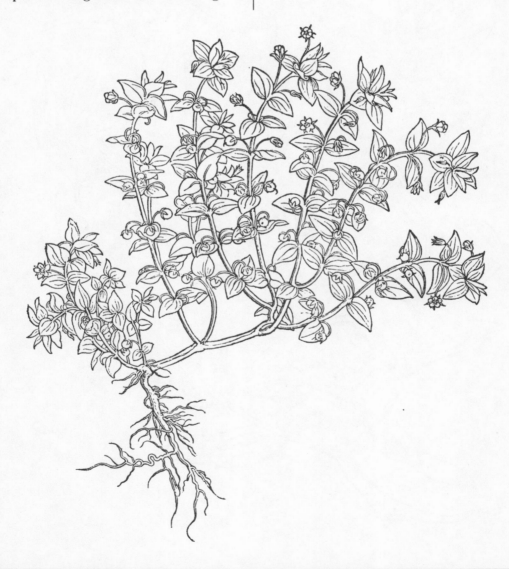

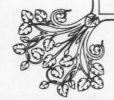
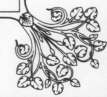

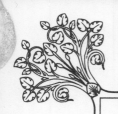

WRINKLES

Wrinkles should merely indicate where smiles have been.
MARK TWAIN, *PUDDIN'HEAD WILSON'S NEW CALENDAR*

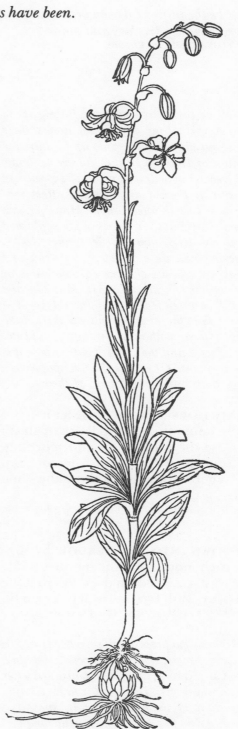

Wouldn't it save hours of fretting, if we could be so philosophical when we first discover those dreaded wrinkles. Wrinkles appear faster on dried-out skin, so the constant use of moisturizers will discourage them. But, if you already have them, here are a couple of 'wrinkle removers'.

TO TAKE AWAY WRINKLES: Take two ounces of the powder of myrrh, lay it in a small fire shovel till it be red hot, then take a mouthful of white wine and let it fall gently upon the myrrh, which will smoke up, when you must hold your face over it till the whole is washed, it will have a wonderful effect; but if that is too painful, you may cover your face with a cloth.
THE COMPLEAT VERMIN KILLER AND USEFUL POCKET GUIDE, DUBLIN, 1778

A SIMPLE BALSAMIC WATER WHICH REMOVES WRINKLES: Take barley water, strained through a piece of fine linen cloth and drop into it a few drops of Balm of Gilead, shake the bottle for several hours until the Balsam is entirely incorporated with the water which is known by the turbid milky appearance of the mixture. This greatly improves the complexion and preserves the bloom of youth. If used only once a day, it takes away wrinkles and gives the skin a surprising lustre. Before the fluid is used, the face should be washed clean with rain water.
OLD PAMPHLET ON COSMETICS, ONTARIO ARCHIVES

No deity can delay the wrinkles
HORACE, 23 BC

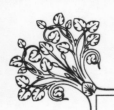

Freckles

Four be the things I'd been better without,
Love, curiosity, freckles and doubt
DOROTHY PARKER, *INVENTORY*

It may be considered cute for little girls to have a sprinkling of freckles across their noses, but they usually grow up to share the opinion of Dorothy Parker. Today we know that freckles appear as a result of exposure to the sun and wind and usually affect red-haired or fair-skinned people. However, this is how The Farmer's Advocate *explained freckles to its readers in September, 1875. 'Freckles indicate a defective digestion and consist in deposits of some carbonaceous or fatty matter beneath the scarf skin. The diet should be attended to and should be of a nature that the kidneys will do their duty. Daily bathing with much friction should not be neglected and the Turkish baths taken if it is convenient.' Of course the newspaper had suggestions on how to get rid of them.*

GRATE HORSERADISH FINE, let it stand a few hours in buttermilk, then strain and use the wash night and morning. Or squeeze the juice of a lemon into half a goblet of water and use the same way.
THE FARMER'S ADVOCATE, LONDON, ONTARIO, SEPT. 1875

GO DOWN INTO THE MEADOW by sunrise each morning in the month of May and wash your face in the dew from the grass, or, wash face in fresh buttermilk.
THE CANADA FARMER, TORONTO, 1 MAY 1865

This whimsical piece of advice was printed in the very practical and informative paper, The Canada Farmer, *in response to a letter from a young girl. It is similar to Dr Chase's suggestion to wash the face in sparkling morning dew to ensure a beautiful complexion. The practice of collecting May dew for medical and beauty cures has a long tradition. We find this comment in Samuel Pepys' diary in 1667: 'To Woolwich ... and so to gather Maydew.' And Francis Bacon noted in 1626. 'I suppose that he that would gather the best Maydew, for medicine, should gather it from the hills.' These esteemed gentlemen may have been following the explicit instruction of Sir Hugh Platt, published in 1609.*

HOW TO GATHER AND CLARIFIE MAYDEAWE: when there hath fallen no rain the night before, then with a cleane and large sponge, the next morning you may gather the same from sweet hearbs, grasse or corne; straine your deawe and expose it to the sunne in glasses covered with paper or parchment prickt full of holes, strain it often, continuing in the sunne and in a hole place till the same grow white and cleere, which may require the best part of the summer.
SIR HUGH PLATT, *DELIGHTS FOR LADIES,* 1609

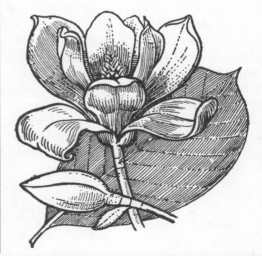

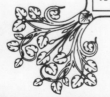

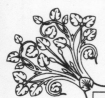

In Delights for Ladies, *Sir Hugh recommended these treatments for removing spots and freckles.*

TO TAKE AWAY FRECKLES IN THE FACE: Wash your face in the wane of the moone with a sponge, morning and evening with the distilled water of Elder leaves, letting the same drie into the skinne. Your water must be distilled in May. This is of a Travailer who hath cured himself thereby.

TO TAKE AWAY SPOTS AND FRECKLES: The sappe that issueth out of a Birch tree in great abundance, being opened in March or Aprill, with a receiver of glass set under the boring thereof to receive the same, doth perform the same most excellently and maketh the skin very cleare. This sap will dissolve pearl, a secret not known to many.

Albertus Magnus also expounded the virtues of 'dew' for removing freckles.

WHEN PERSONS HAVE FRECKLES, catch the dew that settles on wheat, mix with rosewater and oil of lilies. With this water wash the face. It drives all freckles away and adds to the beauty of the face by improving the complexion. *ALBERTUS MAGNUS OR EGYPTIAN SECRETS*

Here is a variety of freckle cures using mainly natural ingredients.

A MEAL OF OATS boiled with vinegar and applied, taketh away freckles and spots in the face and other parts of the body.
An ointment being made with Cowslips, taketh away spots and wrinkles of the skin, sun-burning and freckles, and adds beauty exceedingly.
NICHOLAS CULPEPER, *THE ENGLISH PHYSICIAN* 1652

BITTER ALMONDS AND BARLEY FLOUR: Bitter almonds and barley flour, in equal parts, applied in the form of paste will remove freckles.
THE PEOPLE'S HOME MEDICAL BOOK, CLEVELAND, 1916

A WASH TO REMOVE FRECKLES: Barley water, made thick, two fluid ounces, distilled water of bean-flowers, two fluid ounces; spirits of wine, two fluid ounces. The pickled or tanned skin to be washed often with this preparation.
THE HOUSEHOLD BOOK OF PRACTICAL RECEIPTS, LONDON, 1871

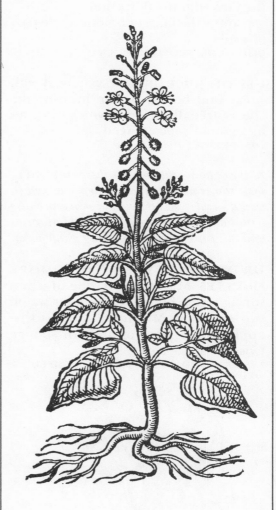

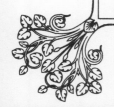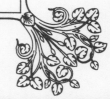

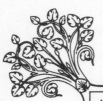

A WATER TO PREVENT FRECKLES OR BLOTCHES IN THE FACE: Take wild cucumber roots and narcissus roots, of each an equal amount; dry them in the shade and reduce them to a very fine powder, putting them afterwards into very strong French Brandy, with which wash the face till it begins to itch, and then wash it with cold water. This method must be repeated every day till a perfect cure is obtained, which will soon happen for, this water has a slight caustic property and of course, must remove all spots on the face.

OR, boil ivy leaves in wine and foment the face with the decoction.

OR, apply the juice of onions to the part affected.

OLD PAMPHLET ON COSMETICS, N.D.

USE THE JUICE OF LEMONS mixed with sugar and borax; or the juice of the cherry-tree dissolved in vinegar; or an infusion of cabbage seed.

THE DOMESTIC PHYSICIAN, 1845

At the opposite extreme are these cures using some rather nasty sounding chemicals, which would simply take off layers of skin and cause irritation. Muriatic acid is hydrochloric acid, and salt petre is used in making gunpowder.

DR KITTOE'S WASH TO REMOVE FRECKLES: Muriatic acid, one drachm; spring water, one pint; lavender water, two drachms. Mix for a lotion to be applied on a piece of linen or sponge twice or thrice a day.

THE HOUSEHOLD BOOK OF PRACTICAL RECEIPTS, LONDON, 1871

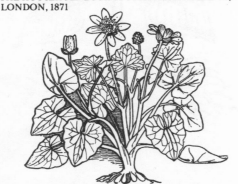

RUB THEM TWICE DAILY with a piece of salt petre, moistened by touching it in water.

DR CHASE'S RECIPES, 1892 EDITION

TAKE ONE DRACHM OF CAUSTIC POTASH and dissolve it in one quart of water, add one ounce of pure almond oil and shake well. Add a tablespoon of this to some soft water and wash the face with it.

THE FARMER'S ADVOCATE, LONDON, ONTARIO, 1883

FOR THE BENEFIT OF YOUNG PERSONS affected with freckles, we would say, that powdered nitre moistened with water, applied to the face night and morning will soon remove all traces of them.

NEWSPAPER CLIPPING FROM CANADIAN PIONEER DIARY

These folk remedies certainly are not harmful. Whether they have any effect on freckles is another question.

TEXAS REMEDIES:
• Take a glass of urine and mix it with a tablespoon of good vinegar. Add a pinch of salt. Let it set for twenty-four hours, then put it on the freckled skin and leave it for one half-hour. Rinse with plain cold water.
• Cut a cucumber in two and rub it on the face.
• Stay indoors for three days. Then go outside and cover the freckles with mud. When the mud dries, wash it off and the freckles will be gone.
• Washing the face with a wet diaper will remove freckles.
• Catch a live frog and rub it over the face.
• Bathe the freckled area in warm beer.
• Apply horse manure pack to the face.
• Rub a freshly cut potato on the freckles.

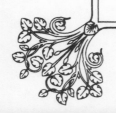

TO TAK AWAY FRECKLES AND TO MAK A FEAR SKIN: Anoint ye face with ye blood of a hare.
DORSET FOLK REMEDY, 17TH C.

TO REMOVE FRECKLES, wash your face with melon rind.
To cure freckles, go to a stone and step over it three times backwards and then three times forward.
KENTUCKY SUPERSTITIONS, 1920

PUT SAP from a grape vine on them.
Put stump water on them.
APPALACHIAN REMEDIES

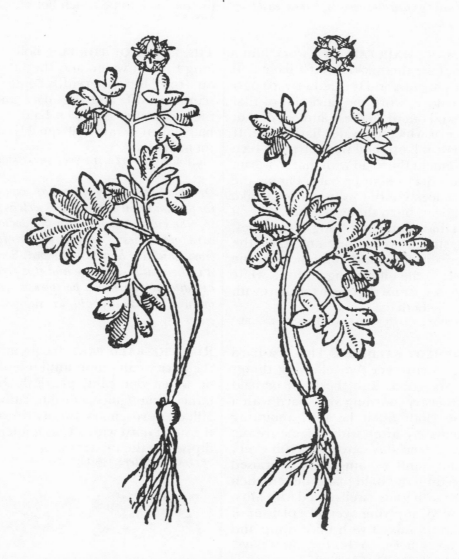

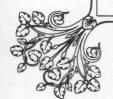
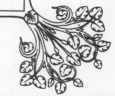

Hair

BALDNESS

There's no time for a man to recover his hair that grows bald by nature.
SHAKESPEARE, *THE COMEDY OF ERRORS*

If everyone shared this pessimistic opinion with Shakespeare, there would not be any baldness cures. The following remedies did not always guarantee results, but at least they offered hope.

IF A MAN'S HAIR FALL OFF, work him a salve. Take the mickle wolf's bane and viper's bugloss and the netherward part of burdock, work the salve out of that wort and out of all these and out of that butter of which no water hath come. If the hair fall off, boil the polypody fern and fement the head with that so warm. In case that a man be bald, Plinius the mickle leech saith this leechdom. 'Take dead bees, burn them to ashes, add oil upon that, seethe very long over gledes, then strain, wring out and take the leaves of willow, pound them, pour the juice into the oil; boil again for a while on gledes, strain them, smear therewith after the bath.'
LEECH BOOK OF BALD, 10TH C. ANGLO-SAXON CURE

TO REMEDY BALDNESS: This is a hard thing to cure yet the following things are very good. Rub the head or bald places every morning very hard with a coarse cloth till it be red, anointing immediately after with Bear's grease; when fifteen days are past, rub every morning and evening with a braised onion until the Bald places be red, then anoint with honey well mixed with Mustard seed, applying over all a plaister of laudanum mixed with mice dung and powder of bees, do this for thirty days.
WILLIAM SALMON, POLYGRAPHICES

BRANDY AND SALT were supposed to have the power of restoring the hair, though sheep dip was held by some in the outback to be much better.
AUSTRALIAN CURE

THE ROOTS OF THE ELM boiled for a long time in water, and the fat arising on the top thereof, being clean scummed off, and the place anointed therewith that is grown bald, and the hair fallen away, will quickly restore them again.
NICHOLAS CULPEPER, *THE ENGLISH PHYSICIAN*, 1652

Dr Chase frequently offered an explanation for the condition or ailment as well as providing the cure. According to the doctor, 'The cause of baldness is defect in the hair follicles, from which the hair is developed. Sometimes it is the result of disease and it is frequently hereditary. Those who perspire much about the head are usually bald.' He suggested these cures.

RUB THE BALD PART frequently with the juice of an onion until it looks red; or water, one pint; pearlash, half an ounce; onion juice, one gill; rum, half a gill; oil of rosemary, twenty drops. Rub the head hard with a rough linen towel dipped in the mixture.
DR CHASE'S RECIPES, 1880 EDITION

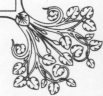

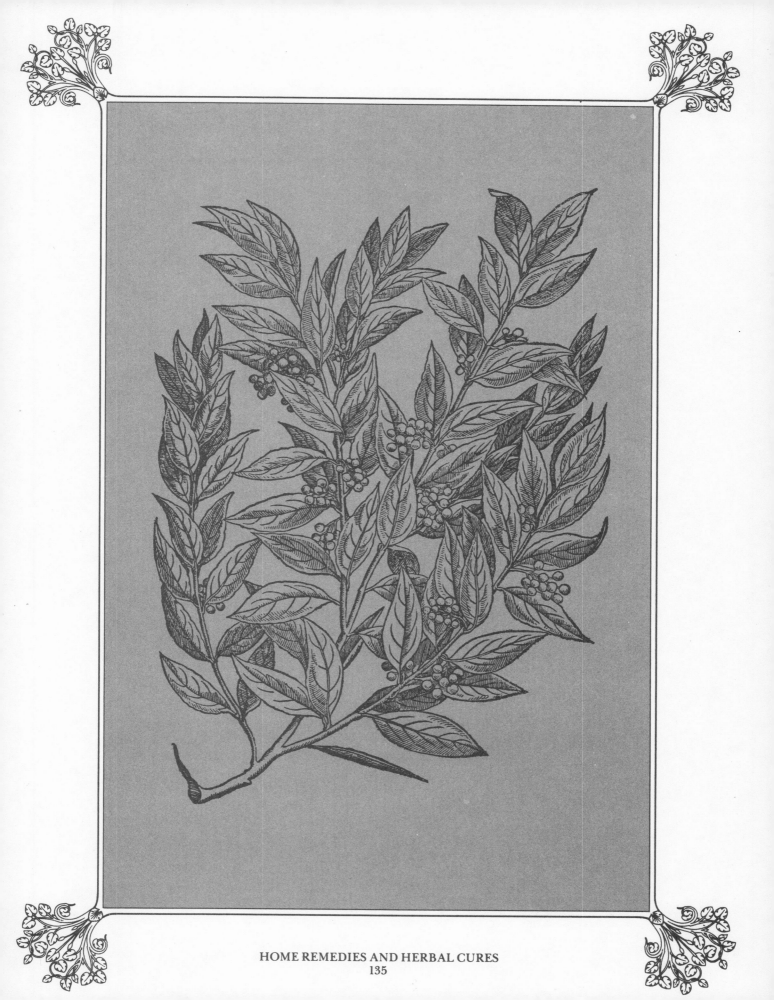

As usual, the Texans resorted to cow manure.

• Smear your head with fresh cow manure.
• Rub your head daily with axle grease and cod liver oil.
• Obtain some mud from a river which has been out for two months. Soak the mud in water for ten minutes and salt well. Place the mud on your head.
TEXAN REMEDIES

Following the proverb that 'prevention is better than cure,' here are a couple of ways to keep your hair. For, as Oliver Herford said, 'a hair in the head is worth two in the brush.'

TO PREVENT THE HAIR FALLING OFF: Wash the head once a day with good old Jamaica rum.
U.S. PRACTICAL RECEIPT BOOK, 1844

THREE OUNCES OF TARTARIC ACID, a few drops of lemon juice in six ounces of soft water, with this wet the head two or three times a week. The skin will be soft and the hair firm.
FARMER'S DIRECTORY AND HOUSEKEEPER'S ASSISTANT, TORONTO, 1851

If you're already bald, take heart. Albertus Magnus offered two remedies to 'cause the hair to grow wherever you wish.'

Take milk of a slut and saturate therewith the spot wherever the hair is desired to grow. Probatum est.
OR
Take dog's milk and paint the spot therewith, wherever you wish to have the hair grow. It will surely grow.

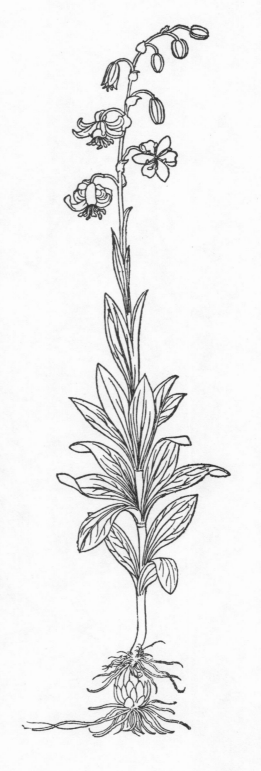

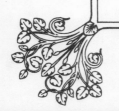
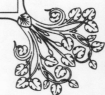

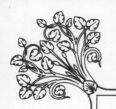

DEPILATORIES

While some people don't have enough hair, others have too much to suit them. Here's a selection of remedies to get rid of hair from various parts of the body.

TO REMOVE HAIR FROM THE NOSTRILS: Take some very fine and clean wood ashes, dilute them with a little water and with the finger apply some of the mixture within the nostrils. The hair will be removed without the least pain.
THE FAMILY MANUAL, NEW YORK, 1845

A SIMPLE DEPILATORY: Oil of Walnuts frequently rubbed on a child's forehead will prevent the hair from growing on that part.
OLD PAMPHLET ON COSMETICS, *ONTARIO ARCHIVES*

TO REMOVE SUPERFLUOUS HAIR: Saturate the part well with fine oil. In about an hour, wipe it off; then take finely powdered quick lime, one ounce, powdered orpiment, one dram, mix with white of egg, and apply with a small brush.
DR CHASE'S RECIPES, 1880 EDITION

Orpiment, also known as yellow arsenic, is a bright yellow mineral substance.

A REMARKABLE PASSAGE FROM THE BOOK OF ALBERTUS MAGNUS: It says: If you burn a large frog to ashes and mix the ashes with water, you will obtain an ointment that will, if put on any place covered with hair, destroy the hair and prevent it from growing again.
THE LONG LOST FRIEND, 1856

TO MAKE THE EYEBROWS APPEAR BEAUTIFUL: Mix with the blood of a young cock, half an ounce of emmets eggs, the same quantity of gum of ivy, colsponia and burnt leeches; when they are all dissolved and mingled, put them close up in a wide mouthed glass, then take a pencil, dip it in and touch with it those parts of the eyebrows where you want the hair to come off.
THE COMPLEAT VERMIN KILLER AND USEFUL POCKET COMPANION, DUBLIN 1778

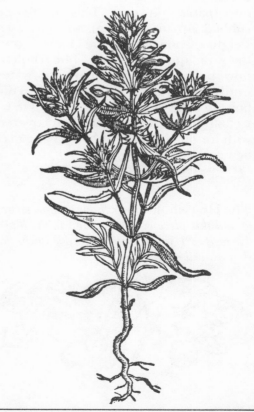

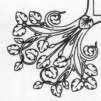

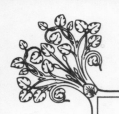

DYES

"Troubles have brung these grey hairs and this premature balditude."
MARK TWAIN, *THE ADVENTURERS OF HUCKLEBERRY FINN*

If troubles have 'brung' you grey hairs, here are two possible remedies.

TO PREVENT GREY HAIR: Take four ounces of butternut hulls, infuse them in a quart of water for an hour and then add one half ounce of copperas. The hair should be brushed with the solution every few days.
ONTARIO PIONEER REMEDY

BLACK DYE FOR HAIR: Bruised nutgalls, half a pound; to be boiled in olive oil until they are soft. They are then to be dried on a stone and reduced to impalpable powder. This is to be rubbed up in a mortar with its own weight of powdered vine charcoal and the same quantity of salt. The whole is now boiled in three quarts of water until a greasy black sediment falls to the bottom. This is the dye. The hair is to be well anointed with it and then covered with an oil-skin cap. When dry, it may be brushed out.
THE HOUSEHOLD BOOK OF PRACTICAL RECEIPTS,
LONDON, 1871

The Household Book thought it necessary to add this piece of information to the black dye recipe: 'Unfortunately, this dye stains the skin as well as the hair.'

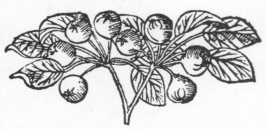

The Family Oracle made it very clear that 'light eyebrows' were a liability to be corrected as quickly as possible. 'Very light eyebrows, indeed, impart to the countenance a sort of babyish vacony and simpletonism which must always distract from the influence of the most beautiful features, or the finest eyes.' The Oracle gave the following recipe for darkening the eyebrows and thus avoiding looking like a simpleton.

WASH FOR DARKENING THE EYEBROWS: Dissolve in one ounce of distilled water, one drachm of sulphate of iron, add one ounce of gum water, a teaspoonful of eau de Cologne. Mix and after having wetted the eyebrows with the aromatic tincture of galls, apply the wash with a camel hair pencil.

Burn a clove in the flame of a wax candle, dip it in the juice of elder berries and apply it to the eyebrows.
THE FAMILY ORACLE OF HEALTH, ECONOMY, MEDICINE AND GOOD LIVING, LONDON, 1825

While you're darkening the eyebrows, you may as well do the eyelashes too.

TO BLACKEN THE EYELASHES: The simplest preparation for this purpose, are the juice of elderberries, burnt cork and cloves burnt at the candle. Another means is, to take the black of frankincense, resin and mastic. This black will not come off with perspiration.
THE FAMILY MANUAL, NEW YORK, 1845

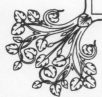
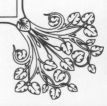

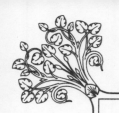

SHAMPOOS AND DANDRUFF TREATMENTS

No matter what colour, hair is not attractive if dirty or full of dandruff. Here are some old-fashioned shampoos and dandruff cures.

DANDRUFF: Take one pint of alcohol and a tablespoon of castor oil, mix together in a bottle by shaking them well for a few minutes, then scent it with a few drops of lavender.
THE CANADA FARMER, TORONTO, 1 JUNE 1866

TAKE GLYCERINE, four ounces, tincture of cantharides, five ounces, bayrum, four ounces, water, two ounces. Mix, and apply once a day and rub well down the scalp.
THE NEW COOK BOOK, 1906

Cantharide is another name for Spanish Fly, which is more usually mentioned as an aphrodisiac.

SHAMPOO: Half an ounce of gum camphor dissolved in two quarts of hot water, one ounce of glycerine, half an ounce of borax. Shake well and wash your hair. Brush the hair and then rinse in clean water. It cleanses the head and gives to the hair a beautiful glossy look.
THE FARMER'S ADVOCATE, LONDON, ONTARIO, NOVEMBER, 1876.

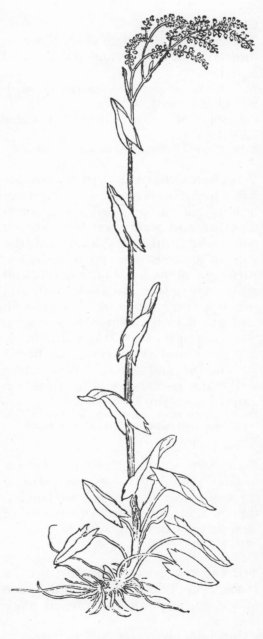

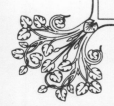

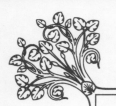

Hands and Nails

CHAPPED HANDS:
To prevent: Wash them with flour of mustard. Or, in bran and water boiled together.
To Cure: Wash with soft soap mixed with red sand (Tried)
Or, wash them in sugar and water (Tried)
REVEREND JOHN WESLEY, *PRIMITIVE PHYSICK*, 1747

TO CLEAN AND SOFTEN THE HANDS: Set half a pint of milk over the fire, and put into it half a quartern of almonds blanched and beaten very fine, when it boils, take it off and thicken with the yolk of an egg; then set it on again, stirring it all the while both before and after the egg is in; then take it off and stir in a small spoonful of Sweet Oil; and put it in a Gallipot. It will keep about five or six days. Take a bit as big as a Wallnut and rub about your hands and the Dirt and Soil will rub off and it will make them very soft. Draw on gloves just as you have used it.
THE COMPLETE FAMILY PIECE AND COUNTRY GENTLEMAN AND FARMER'S BEST GUIDE, LONDON, 1741

FACE AND HAND LOTION: Take on quarter pound of honey and warm it through; add half a pound lanolin, then beat in one quarter of a pound of almond oil. Cool and bottle.
NEW ENGLAND SIMPLE

TO TAKE STAINES OUT OF ONE'S HANDS PRESENTLY: This is done with the juice of sorrell, washing the stayned place therein.
SIR HUGH PLATT, *DELIGHTS FOR LADIES*, 1609

TO REMOVE THE COLOR OF NAILS THAT HAVE BECOME BLACK BY BRUISING: Mix two scruples of flour of sulphur, with two drachms of capon's grease, and the same quantity of oil of chammomile; put to it a drachm of oil of roses and a few grains of cummin seed, mix the whole together and lay a small bit on leather which must be put to the nails when you go to bed.
THE COMPLEAT VERMIN KILLER AND USEFUL POCKET GUIDE, DUBLIN, 1778

EMOLLIENT FOR THE NAILS: is made in the following way.
Enough melted white vasoline to fill a tablespoon. Put it into a deep bottle, beat it, and while it is hot, stir into it a lump of spermacetti as big as half a walnut. Add to it six drops of perfume and set it away to cool.
MOORE'S ALMANACK LONDON, 1912

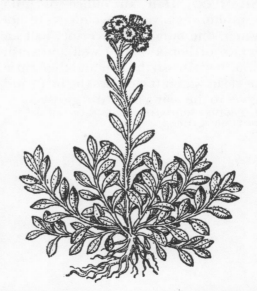

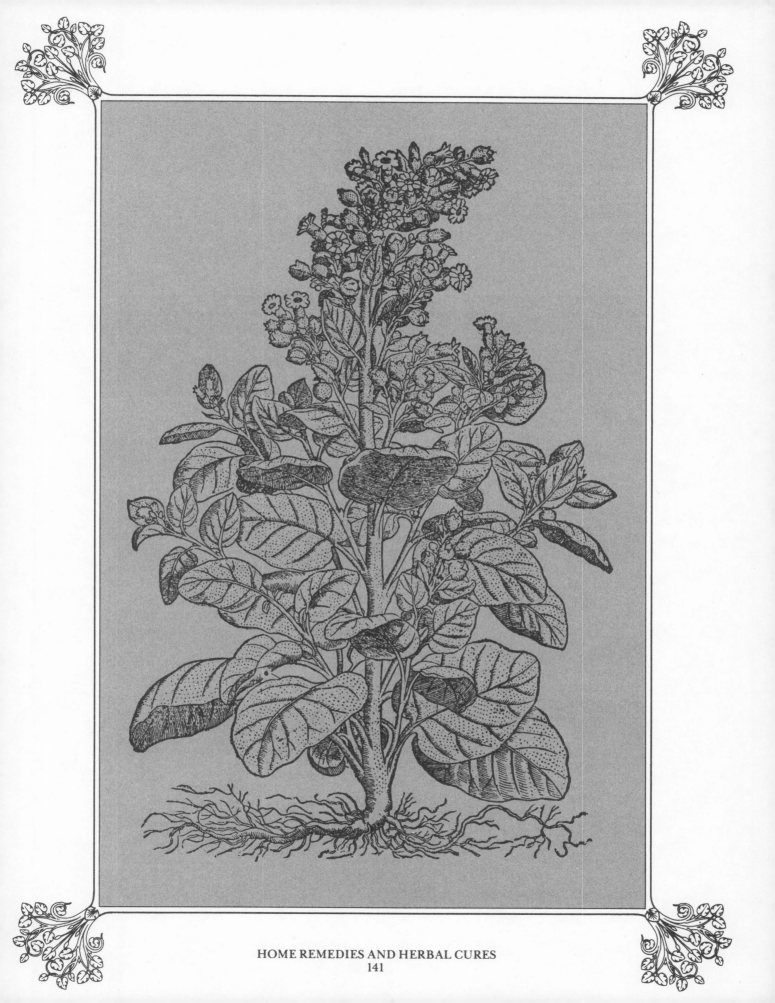

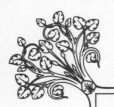

Lips

O, how ripe in show
Thy lips, those kissing cherries, tempting grow
SHAKESPEARE, *A MIDSUMMER NIGHT'S DREAM*

These early lip salves use similar ingredients to soften and redden the lips. Alkanet, an herb cultivated in central and southern Europe, gives a deep red colour when mixed with oily substances. Spermacetti comes from the sperm whale, which in the days of extensive whaling, was a popular ingredient in the preparation of medicines, cosmetics and candles.

A FINE LIP SALVE: Take two ounces of Virgin's wax, two ounces of hog's lard, half an ounce of spermacetti, one ounce of oil of sweet almonds, two ounces of balsam of Peru, two drams of alkenet root, cut small, six new raisons shred small, a little fine sugar, simmer them all together a little while, then strain it off into little pots. It is the finest lip salve in the world.
THE ART OF COOKERY MADE PLAIN AND EASY BY A LADY, 1760

KITTOE'S SCARLET LIP SALVE: Take hog's lard washed in rose water, half a pound, red and damask rose leaves bruised, quarter of a pound, work them well together in a mortar and let them lay two days; then melt the lard, and strain it, add to the lard the same quantity of rose leaves, let them lay two days as before, simmer in a water-bath, and strain, stirring in five or six drops of otto of roses. Put into pots or boxes for use.
THE HOUSEHOLD BOOK OF PRACTICAL RECEIPTS, LONDON, 1871

The use of lip salves and all other beautifying cosmetics came to an abrupt end in England in 1770. They had become enormously popular with all classes of women. Suddenly, the menfolk decided that the use of cosmetics was an issue of enough importance to warrant an Act of Parliament. Their fears and concerns are clearly stated in the following edict: 'That all women of whatever age, rank, profession or degree, whether virgin maid or widow, that shall from and after such Act impose upon, seduce and betray into matrimony any of His Majesty's subjects by means of scent, paints, cosmetic washes, artificial teeth, false hair, Spanish wool, iron stays, hoops, high-heeled shoes or bolstered hips, shall incur the penalty of the law now in force against witchcraft and like misdemeanours, and that married upon conviction, shall stand null and void.'

The next innocuous suggestion probably would not have offended any of His Majesty's subjects.

TO TAKE OFF THE HEAT AND ROUGHNESS OF THE SKIN, ESPECIALLY ON THE LIPS: Anoint the part affected with fresh (or at least not too stale) Cream.
THE COMPLETE FAMILY PIECE AND COUNTRY GENTLEMAN AND FARMER'S BEST GUIDE, LONDON 1741

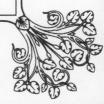

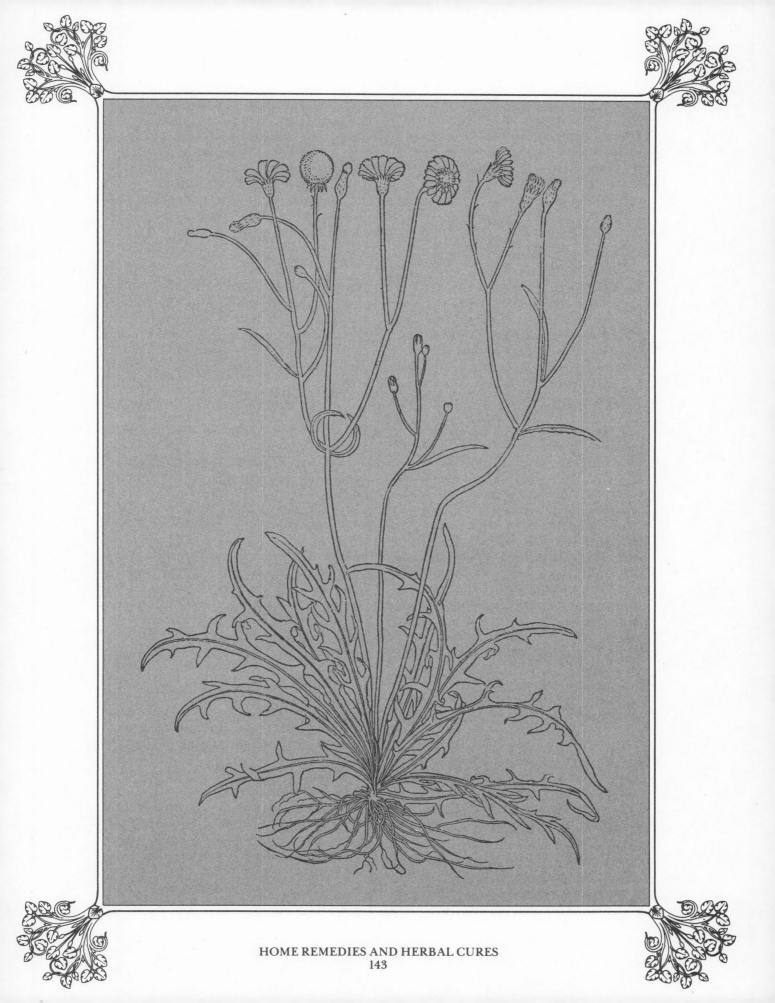

Perfumes

All the perfumes of Arabia will not sweeten this little hand.
SHAKESPEARE, *MACBETH*

Perfumes have been with us since the days of the ancient civilizations and recipes and techniques of perfume-making were coveted by less advanced societies. All the eastern cultures, the Babylonians, Chinese, Syrians, Indians, Persians, Assyrians, had a sophisticated proficiency with scents. The Egyptian civilization was probably the first to practise distillation for making perfumes, and Cleopatra went to the extremes of having her mattress stuffed with roses and the floors of her palace covered eighteen inches deep in rose petals. It was from the Egyptians that the Greeks and Romans acquired the habit of anointing their bodies. In fact, the Romans became so obsessed with perfume that a law was passed in 565 restraining the use of 'exotics' for private use. In the early Christian era, aromatic oils were used for anointing and embalming the body.

In England, interest in perfumes reached its climax during the reign of Elizabeth I, who blended and invented scents herself in the royal still-room just like other ladies of the manor. Often Queen Elizabeth gave her recipes away to other reigning sovereigns. Here are two of her Majesty's personal recipes taken from the book A Queen's Delight, *1671.*

QUEEN ELIZABETH'S PERFUME: Take eight spoonfuls of compound water, the weight of two pence in fine powder of sugar, and boil it on hot embers and coals, softly, and half an ounce of sweet Marjoram, dried in the sun, the weight of two pence of the powder of Benjamin. This perfume is very sweet and good for the time.

KING EDWARD'S PERFUME: Take twelve spoonfuls of right Red Rose Water, the weight of six pence in fine powder of Sugar, and boil it on hot embers and coals softly, and the house will smell as though it were full of Roses; but you must burn the sweet cyprus wood before, to take away the gross airs.

Perfumes were believed to be antiseptic and purifying, and herbs were strewn over the floors to ward off the plague and other germs.

Even Sir Walter Raleigh, adventurer and favourite of the Queen, developed an interest in perfume-making. After Elizabeth's successor, James I, banished Sir Walter to the Tower of London for 13 years, he is said to have set up a laboratory and practised distillation in his closet-sized cell. His recipe for a perfumed cordial was believed to contain some secret herb which he had discovered on his expedition to Guyana, but as we can see, it was rather straightforward and simple.

A CORDIAL WATER OF SIR WALTER RALEIGH: Take a gallon of Strawberries and put them in a pint of aqua vitae, let them stand so four or five days, strain them gently out and sweeten the water as you please with fine Sugar or else with perfume.
A QUEEN'S DELIGHT, 1671

Aqua vitae is actually brandy.

Continuing on with the regal theme, here are two recipes for perfumes for Queen Victoria and her Consort, Albert.

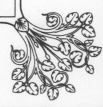

THE QUEEN'S OWN PERFUME: Essences of cloves and bergamotte, of each three quarters of a drachm; neroli, about a drachm; essence of musk, half an ounce; eau de rose, spirit of tuberose, and the strongest spirits of wine, of each half a pint; spirits of jasmine and cassia, of each one pint; dissolve the essences in the spirit of wine, then add the other spirits and when well mixed, add the rose water.
THE HOUSEHOLD BOOK OF PRACTICAL RECEIPTS,
LONDON, 1871

PRINCE ALBERT'S OWN PERFUME: Ambergris, half an ounce; musk, three drachms; lump sugar, two drachms; grind together in a Wedgewood-ware mortar, add of oil of cloves, ten drops; of true balsam of Peru, twenty drops, and the essence of jasmine or tuberose, a sufficient quantity to convert it into a perfectly smooth paste; then put it into a bottle with rectified spirits of wine, one quart. Observe, before adding the whole of the last, to rinse the mortar out well with it, that nothing may be lost. Lastly, digest for six or eight weeks. The result will be a remarkably fine product. A very small quantity added to lavendar water, eau de cologne, toothpowder, washballs and a hogshead of claret communicates a delicious fragrance.
THE HOUSEHOLD BOOK OF PRACTICAL RECEIPTS,
LONDON, 1871

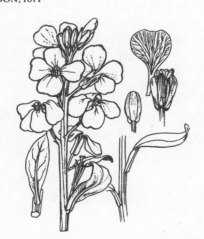

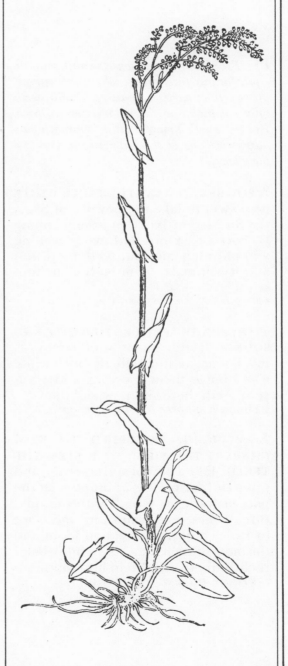

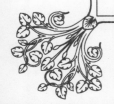

Teeth

Hot things, sharp things, sweet things, cold things,
All rot the teeth and make them look like old things.
BENJAMIN FRANKLIN, *POOR RICHARD'S ALMANACK*, 1734

Ben Franklin's rhyme was the unfortunate truth for our forefathers, who lived without the benefit of modern dentistry. Usually teeth only got attention when they were aching. But those with a more positive approach may have tried one of the following to preserve their teeth.

A POWDER TO MAKE THE TEETH WHITE AND SWEET: Take the powder of Sage, the Shaving of Ivory, put them among ye juice of lemons and every evening and morning rub your teeth therewith and it will make them both white and sweet.
A BOOK OF SIMPLES, LONDON C. 1750

TO KEEP THE TEETH BOTH WHITE AND SOUND: Take a quantity of honey, as much vinegar and halfe so much white wine, boyle them together and wash your teeth therewith now and then.
SIR HUGH PLATT, *DELIGHTS FOR LADIES*, 1609

A MEDICINE PRESCRIB'D TO KING CHARLES THE FIRST TO FASTEN THE TEETH: Take a pint of spring-water, and put to it four ounces of brandy: let the patient wash his mouth with the mixture of these every morning and twice or thrice a day besides; and let him in the morning roll for a little while a bit of roch allum to and fro in his mouth.
THE FAMILY MAGAZINE, LONDON, 1741

In his book, The Rules of Christian Manners and Civility, *St. Jean Baptiste de la Salle (1651-1719) gave this advice on dental hygiene. 'It is necessary to clean the teeth frequently, more especially after meals, but not on any account with a pin, or the point of a penknife and it must never be done at the table.' I wonder what he would say to this one recommending a sharp skewer.*

TO CLEAN VERY FOUL SPOTTED TEETH: Make a skewer very sharp at one End, over which wind a Bit of fine Rag, tie it on very hard, and cut it very sharp, that it may be like a fine Pencil for Painting, dip this in Spirit of Salt, take it out immediately, and dip it then into a Cup of Fair Water, in which hold it for a Moment, with this Rag, so carefully wet, rub your Teeth, and take care you do not touch your Lips or Gums; have a Cup of cold Water ready to wash your Mouth, that the Rag has not been dipped in: With this you may make any furr'd teeth as white as Snow; but you must not use it often or carelessly. When they are once thus clean, the Claret wash will preserve them so.
A COLLECTION OF RECEIPTS IN COOKERY, PHYSICK AND SURGERY, LONDON 1749

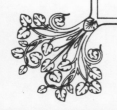
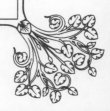

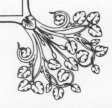

Here's the recipe for the Claret Wash.

A CONSTANT DAILY WASH FOR YOUR TEETH: To one Quart of Claret put an ounce of Bole Armoniack, half an ounce of Myrrh, one dram of Allom, Salt of Vitriol, ten grains, an ounce of Hungary-water, and two ounces of Honey of Roses. When these have stood in a warm Sun or near the Fire for three days, set it by to settle; and pour a spoonful of it into a Teacup of Water, with which wash your Teeth: It preserves them sound and makes them white.
A COLLECTION OF RECEIPTS IN COOKERY PHYSICK AND SURGERY, LONDON 1749

The use of a toothbrush for cleaning teeth is a recent practice. According to Leo Kanner in The Folklore of the Teeth, *the toothbrush has only been around for two to three hundred years. However, the toothpick is at least three thousand years old. It was a common toilet article at the time of the great Roman emperors. And throughout the ages, it has gone by many names, such as toothstick, toothscraper or toothrake. Toothpowders or preparations gained more popularity with the invention of the toothbrush, but were also applied with the finger or a piece of rag. Here are four preparations for cleaning the teeth.*

A NATURAL DENTIFRICE: The common strawberry is a natural dentifrice and its juice without any preparation dissolves the tartareous incrustations on the teeth, and makes the breath sweet and agreeable.
MERCHANT AND FARMER'S ALMANACK, NEW BRUNSWICK, 1855

BURN A SLICE OF BREAD in the oven until it becomes charcoal; then pound in a mortar and sift through a fine muslin cloth.
THE FARMER'S ADVOCATE, LONDON, ONTARIO, APRIL, 1875

ASIATIC DENTIFRICE: Armenian bole, three parts; prepared chalk, two parts, ochre, one part, pumice stone, one part. Reduce to fine powder and sift through lawn. Scent with musk.
U.S. PRACTICAL RECEIPT BOOK, 1844

Armenian bole is a pale reddish earth, used mainly in toothpowders and sometimes given internally for stomach irritations. 'Lawn' refers to a kind of fine linen.

EXCELLENT TOOTHPOWDER: Take any quantity of finely pulverized chalk and twice as much finely pulverized charcoal, make very fine; then add a very little suds made with Castille soap and sufficient spirits of camphor to wet all to a thick paste. Apply with the finger, rubbing thoroughly, and it will whiten the teeth better than any toothpowder you can buy.
DR CHASE'S RECIPES, 1867 EDITION

The peasants of eastern and central Europe have traditionally rinsed out their mouth in the morning with their own urine. If that doesn't appeal to you, perhaps one of these mouthwashes will.

TO CORRECT BAD BREATH: Epsom salts, one drachm, tincture of calumba, two drachms, infusion of roses, one and a half ounces. Mix. To be taken once or twice a week before breakfast.
THE CANADA FARMER, TORONTO 16, MAY 1864

Calumba is a climbing plant indigenous to the forest of Mozambique and it is sometimes used as a mild tonic.

TOOTHWASH: To four ounces of prepared lime-water add a drachm of Peruvian bark; wash the teeth with this water before breakfast and after supper; it will effectually destroy the tartar, and remove the offensive smell from those which are decayed.
BROCKVILLE ALMANAC, 1866.

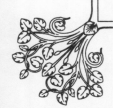

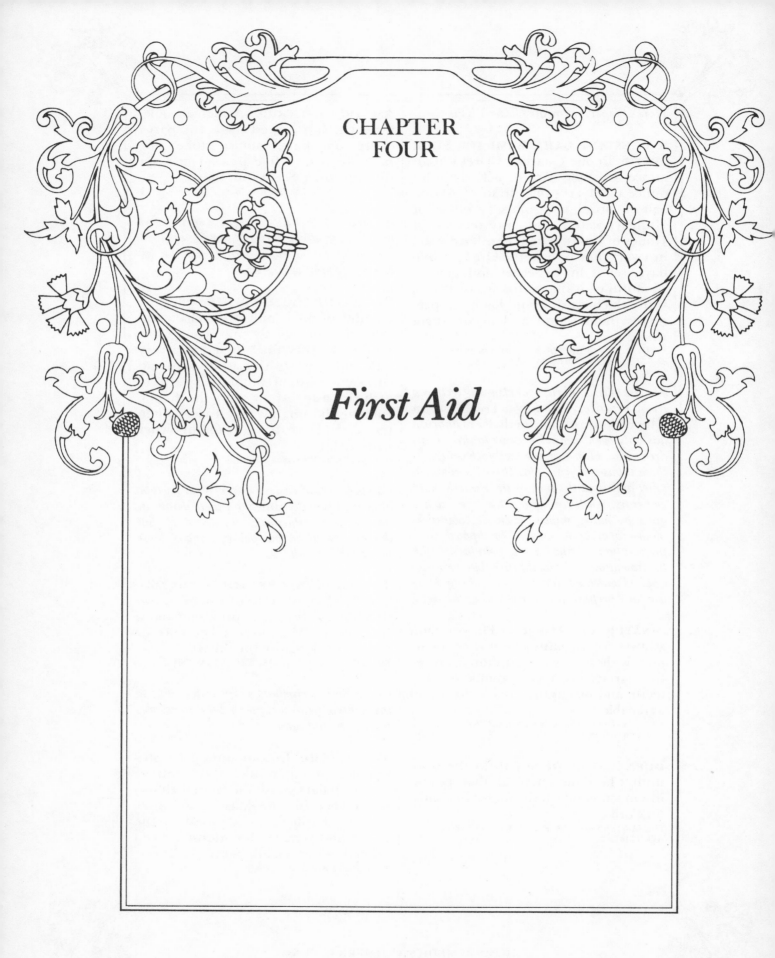

CHAPTER FOUR

First Aid

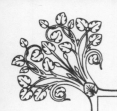

Today there is a special salve or lotion on the market to take care of any little mishap—cuts, scrapes, sprains, sunburn. Our ancestors didn't have the wide variety of products to choose from, although there probably were a couple of patent medicines promising 'wonder cures'. Most of the time, minor accidents were treated with homemade concoctions and children seemed to survive bruised knees and sprained ankles. This section traces some of the first-aid cures used from as early as the 10th century through to recipes from Manor House doctor books and pioneer remedies adapted to the New World and Australia.

Many of the settlers brought their traditional recipes and simply adapted them to use indigenous plants, or copied some of the effective treatments of the natives, such as the North American Indians' use of the dried spores of the puffball to staunch blood. These cures include everything from cobwebs, spiders, dried toads and live pigeons to more practical ingredients such as eggs, bicarbonate of soda, cold water and various herbs.

Some of the ingredients are right there on your kitchen shelf, while others are more difficult to obtain. Even the author of the 10th century Leech Book of Bald *admits that rind from paradise is a scarce commodity. As usual, I have included many of these cures for their entertainment value alone. Others, I am sure you will recognize from childhood days and since you are still around to be reading this book, the remedy must have been effective.*

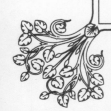
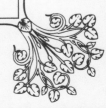

Bites

CAT BITE: For bites from cats, bathe the parts bitten with extract of witch hazel, or if badly bitten wet cotton cloth in the same and bind on and keep parts wet. I have found witch hazel will kill all such poison.
THE PEOPLE'S MEDICAL BOOK, CLEVELAND, OHIO 1916

SPIDER BITE: If bitten by a black widow spider, drink liquor heavily from 3 pm to 7 pm. You won't get drunk, you'll be healed.
APPALACHIAN FOLK REMEDY

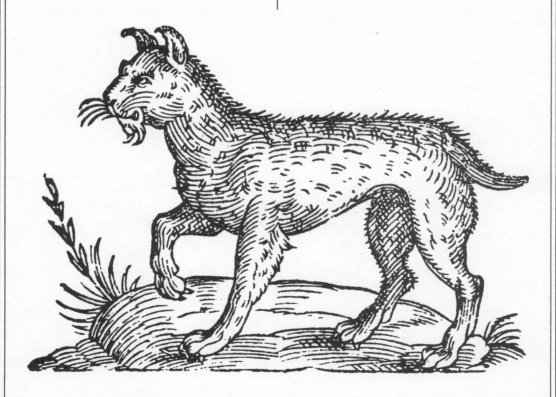

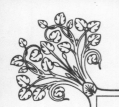

Snake Bites

ADDER BITE: A piece of hazelwood fastened in the shape of a cross should be laid softly on the wound and the following lines twice repeated.

Underneath his hazelin mote,
There's a bragotty worm with speckled throat,
Nine double is he,
Now from eight double to seven double
And from seven double to six double
...and so on to...
And from one double to no double,
No double hath he...
OLD ENGLISH CHARM CURE

AGAINST BITE OF SNAKE: If a man procures and eateth rind, which cometh out of paradise, no venom will damage him. Then said he who wrote this book 'that rind was hard gotten.'
THE LEECH BOOK OF BALD, 10TH C. ANGLO-SAXON MEDICAL MANUSCRIPT

BITE OF VIPER OR RATTLE SNAKE: Apply bruised garlick. Or, rub the place immediately with common oil.
REVEREND JOHN WESLEY, *PRIMITIVE PHYSICK,* 1747

RATTLESNAKE BITES: I know an old physician who called to a boy bitten by a rattlesnake and in the absence of all other remedies, he cured him on the principle that 'The hair of the dog will cure his bite', taking a piece of the snake about two inches long, splitting it upon the back and binding it upon the bite. It cleansed the wound very white and no bad effects were seen from it.
DR CHASE'S RECIPES, 1867 EDITION

CHEW AND SWALLOW, or drink, dissolved in water, alum, the size of a hickory nut.

Put thoroughwort leaves pounded on and keep wetting them with water. If the person is very sick, blue or black, let him drink a little of the juice. Renew the application after two hours.
LADIES INDISPENSABLE ASSISTANT, NEW YORK, 1851

Thoroughwort is also known as boneset, Joe Pye, Indian sage, fever-wort, ague-wort, and as some of the names imply, it was used in North America by both settlers and Indians for fevers.

THE NEGRO CAESAR'S CURE: Take the roots of plantane or hoare-hound (in summer, roots and branches together) a sufficient quantity, bruise them in a mortar, and squeeze out the juice, of which give as soon as possible, one large spoonful, and if he is swell'd you must force it down his throat. This generally will cure: but if the patient finds no relief in an hour after, you may give another spoonful which never fails. To the wound may be applied a leaf of good tobacco, moistened with rum.
THE HOUSEKEEPER'S POCKET-BOOK—EVERYONE THEIR OWN PHYSICIAN, C. 1750

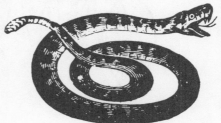

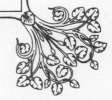

TEXAS REMEDIES:
• Place warm chicken guts on the bite to draw the poison out.
• Take a fresh dead rat and apply the warm meat of the rat to the bite.
• A rattlesnake bite will not be fatal if the victim can cut off the rattler of the snake that bit him.
• Apply kerosene oil in a jar placed upside down over the wound. You will be able to see the green venom being drawn up into the oil.

CARBONATE OF SODA wet and applied externally to the bite of a spider or any venomous creature will neutralize the poisonous effects almost immediately. It acts like a charm in the case of a snake bite. Lean fresh meat will remove the pain of a wasp sting almost instantly and has been recommended for the cure of rattlesnake bites.
THE HEARTHSTONE, PHILADELPHIA, 1883

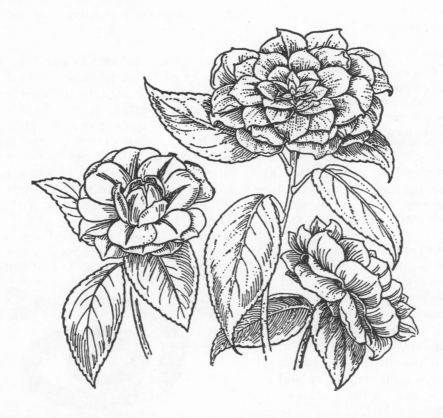

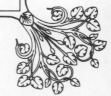

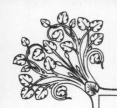

Bruises

THE ROOTS OF SOLOMON'S SEALE stamped while it is fresh and green and applied taketh away in one night, or two at the most, any bruise, blacke or blew spots gotten by fals or women's wilfulness, stumbling upon their hasty husbands' fits or such like.
GERARD'S HERBALL, 1597

FOR A BRUISE OCCASION'D BY A FALL: Take horse dung and sheep suet, of each alike, boil them well together, and apply warm to the part affected as a poultice.
THE FAMILY MAGAZINE, LONDON, 1741

TEXAS REMEDIES:
• Put raw bacon on a bruise to draw out the poison.
• Hold a silver knife or spoon to the bruise. This will keep the spot from turning black and blue and will reduce the swelling.
• Scrape an Irish potato and cook up a poultice from the scrapings. Put this on the bruise.

APPLY A PLASTER of chopped parsley mixed with butter.
REVEREND JOHN WESLEY, PRIMITIVE PHYSICK, 1747

RUB GENTLY with a piece of rag or wool dipped in olive oil, and then cover with a compress saturated with the oil. This gives instant relief and is better than arnica.
THE AUSTRALIAN HOUSEHOLD MANUAL, 1899

TAKE HALF A POUND each of beef tallow, beeswax, rosin and stone pitch and one pint of lard oil. Boil together for half an hour, remove the scum and pour into cups. For use, spread it on kid and apply. It gives immediate relief and it is as good also for domestic animals as it is for man.
THE FARMER'S ADVOCATE, LONDON, ONTARIO FEBRUARY, 1875

MAKE A POULTIS of bran and urine, apply it as hot as you can bear it. If tis very bad repeat it as it cools, and do it as soon as you can, to prevent its swelling, which the air is apt to occasion.
A COLLECTION OF RECEIPTS IN COOKERY, PHYSICK AND SURGERY, 1749

IMMEDIATELY APPLY a cloth, five or six fold, dipped in cold water and new dipped when it grows warm. Or, immediately apply molasses spread on brown paper.
MERCHANT AND FARMER'S ALMANÁCK, NEW BRUNSWICK, 1855

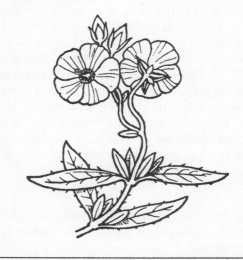

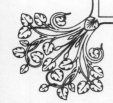
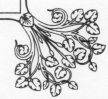

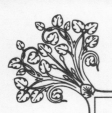

Bruised or Black Eye

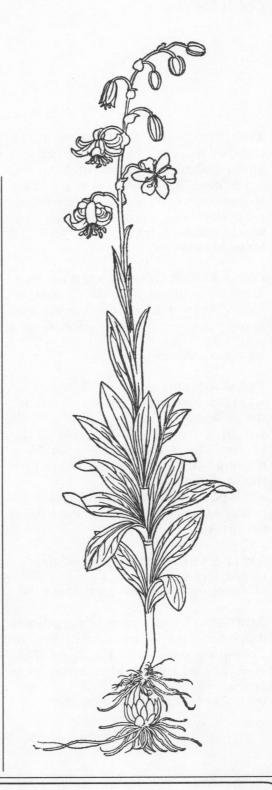

BATHE IT WELL with warm water, then apply a piece of lint soaked in some pure extract of lead. Keep the lint on the eye continually wet with the lotion for three or four hours.
MOORE'S ALMANACK, LONDON 1912

TAKE THE WHITE of an egg, beat it well with cream, dip lint in it and apply to the bruis'd part. It will take out the blood and give ease in a very short time. Renew it once in twelve hours.
THE FAMILY MAGAZINE, LONDON, 1741

BEAT THE LEAVES of eyebright with a rotten apple. Lay it on the eye as a poultice. Repeat it as it grows dry. The juice of the eyebright is as good as the leaves.
THE COMPLETE FAMILY PIECE AND COUNTRY GENTLEMAN AND FARMER'S BEST GUIDE, LONDON, 1741

BOIL A HANDFUL of hyssop leaves in a little water, till they are quite tender, then put them up in linen, and apply it hot to the eye: Tie it on tightly at bedtime, and the eye will next day be quite well. In the original receipt from which the above is taken, it is said, that 'a man who had his thigh terribly bruised by the kick of a horse was cured in a few hours only by a poultice of hyssop leaves cut or minced very small and beaten up with unsalted butter.'
UNIVERSAL RECEIPT BOOK, NEW YORK, 1814

Hyssop, a bushy evergreen herb, will also heal cuts promptly if bruised and applied to the wound.

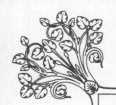

Burns

A BURNING
There came three angels out of the east,
The one brought fire, the other brought frost—
Out Fire; in Frost,
In the Name of The Father, and the Son, And the Holy Ghost. Amen.

TAKE A POUND of rusty bacon, stick it full of oats on every side as it will contain, put a thread through a corner and so hang it on a nail before ye fire and take a blazing stick and sett your bacon of fire and sett a bason of water under it, so let it drop into it, it will be very black when cold. Take it out of ye water and put it in a pott and so anoint ye burns with a plaister.
CURIOUS OLD COOKERY RECEIPTS INCLUDING SIMPLES FOR SIMPLE AILMENTS, LONDON, 1891

MRS HALE'S OINTMENT FOR BURNS OR SCALDS: Take of goose dung, sheep's dung, hen's dung and pidgeon's dung (at the time when pidgeons go a-pecking) an equal quantity of each, boyl them up together in fresh hog's lard or lamb suet.
OLD ENGLISH RECIPE

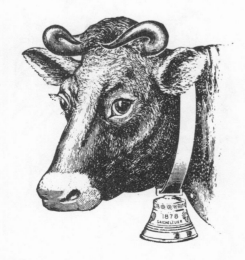

OIL OF BROWN PAPER: Take a piece of the thickest brown paper and dip it in the best salad oil, then set the paper on fire and carefully preserve all the oil that drops, for use. This is said to be an admirable remedy for burns. Oil of writing paper, collected in a similar manner, is often recommended for toothache.
UNIVERSAL RECEIPT BOOK, NEW YORK, 1814

TEXAS REMEDIES:
• Burn a little rabbit fur and beat it to a powder. Mix with linseed oil and rub on the burn.
• For a rope burn, soak the hands in salt water or urine.
• Cut open cactus leaves and put the juice on the burn.
• Hold the burned part near the hot object that burned the victim.
• Go to the lot and make a calf get up and defecate. The feces should be put in a cloth sack which is applied to the burn and left on until the next morning at which time the skin will look like a baby's skin.

TAKE HALF A POUND of deers or mutton sewit pick it clean and melt it. Take a handful of the ivy with white streaks pick it clean and shred it small and take one spoonfull of goosedung. Let it on the fire and boyle it till the leaf will break. Dry and crimp them then strain it and keep for use in a gallypot.
A BOOK OF SIMPLES, LONDON, C. 1750

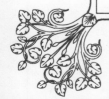
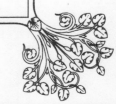

BEESWAX, BURGUNDY PITCH, white pine pitch and rosin, of each a quarter pound; mutton tallow, half a pound, goose oil, one gill, tar, half a gill, mixed and melted together and used as other salves.
DR CHASE'S RECIPES, 1867 EDITION

TAKE LAUREL LEAVES, chop them in hog's grease, strain it and keep it for use.
THE COMPLETE FAMILY PIECE AND COUNTRY GENTLEMAN AND FARMER'S BEST GUIDE, LONDON, 1741

TAKE GREEN VIRGINIA TOBACCO, if you can get it, if not English, bruise it and boyle it in fresh butter, it cures also any cut or green wound, takes out redness and morphew after the small pox. To be made in August.
18TH C. DORSET REMEDY

APPLY THE INNER RIND of elder well mixed with fresh butter. When this is bound on a rag, plunge the part into cold water. This will suspend the pain till the medicine heals. Or, mix lime-water and sweet oil to the thickness of cream and apply it with a feather several times a day. This is a most effectual application.
U.S. PRACTICAL RECEIPT BOOK, 1844

POUND OR PRESS the juice of male ferns and put it on the burnt spots and they will heal very fast. Better yet, however, if you smear the above juice upon a rag and put it on like a plaster.
THE LONG LOST FRIEND, 1856

Culpeper's English Physician *gave another use for male ferns: 'Ferns being burned, the smoak thereof driveth away serpents, gnats and other noisome creatures which in fenny countries do, in the nighttime, trouble the most people lying in their beds with their faces uncovered.'*

APPLY PEACH-TREE LEAVES, the smooth side next to the skin, and bind them on.
BUCKEYE COOKERY, MINNEAPOLIS, 1881

BEAT AN APPLE with salad oil until it is a poultice, pretty soft; bind it on the part and as it dried, lay on fresh.

You must be sure to pare, core and beat your apples well for fear of breaking the skin of the burn. But if the skin be off, there is nothing in nature so sure to take out the fire.
U.S. PRACTICAL RECEIPT BOOK, 1844

BEAT TWO DRACHMS OF SALT with two raw onions, in a mortar and when they are properly mixed, apply some of it to the part affected.
THE COMPLEAT VERMIN KILLER AND USEFUL POCKET COMPANION, DUBLIN, 1778

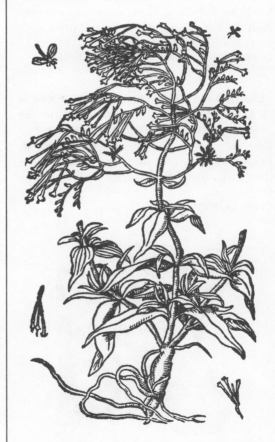

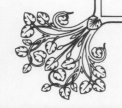
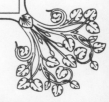

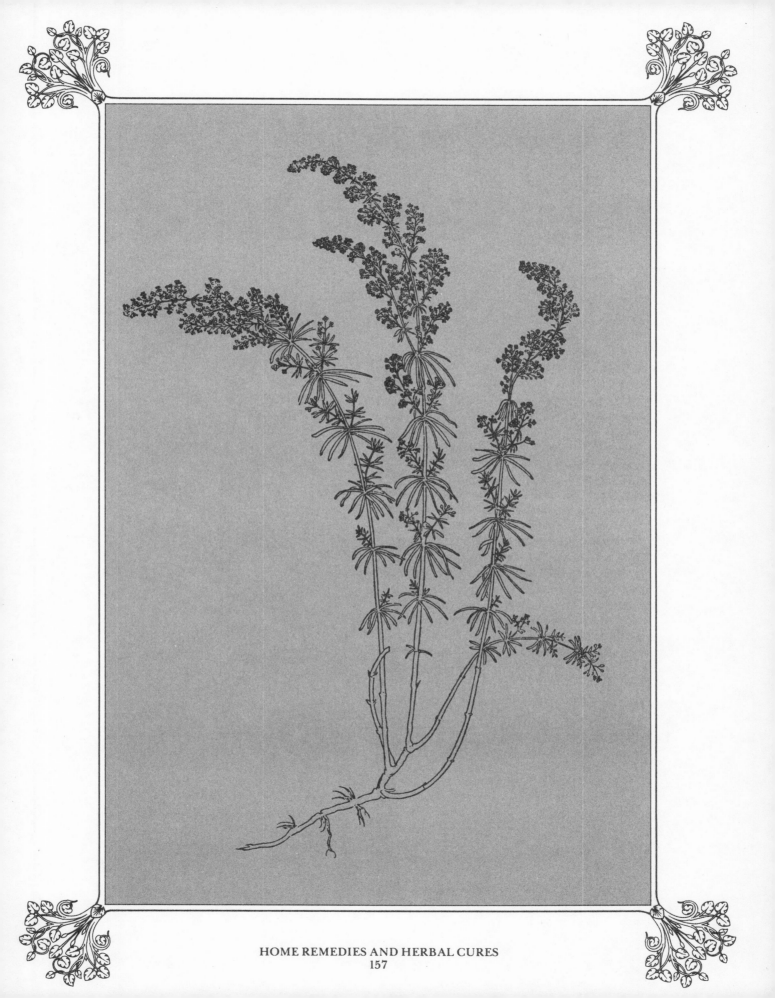

Choking and Other Blockages

SAY THRICE 'I buss the Gorgon's mouth.' This charm repeated thrice nine times will draw out a bone stuck in a man's throat.
LEECHDOMS OF ENGLAND, 10TH C. ANGLO-SAXON REMEDY

TAKE FOUR GRAINS of tartar emetic in warm water and afterwards take the whites of six eggs which will coagulate upon the stomach before the Tartar operates and will envelop either pins or any sharp bones and maybe used with success.
MRS BENJAMIN SMITH, NEWFOUNDLAND, 1841

TO PREVENT CHOKING, break an egg into a cup and give it to the person choking, to swallow. The white of the egg seems to catch around the obstacle and remove it. If one egg does not answer the purpose, try another. The white is all that is necessary.
FARMER'S AND HOUSEKEEPER'S CYCLOPAEDIA, NEW YORK, 1888

ANOTHER EXPEDIENT is to introduce a large goose quill down the throat and then twist it around, for by this means the substance may be disengaged and so pass down into the stomach.
THE HOUSEHOLD BOOK OF PRACTICAL RECEIPTS, LONDON, 1871

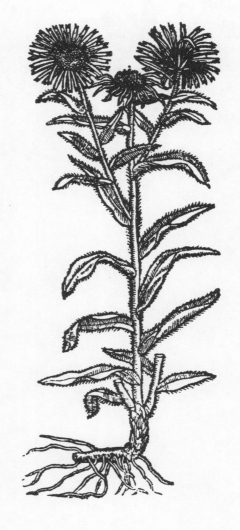

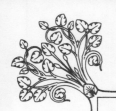

Foreign Objects in the Nose and Ears

SIMPLE METHOD FOR REMOVING INSECTS FROM EARS: Dr. B. F. Kingsley, USA, relates a number of cases where soldiers sleeping on the plains have come to him to have bugs removed from their ears. Accidentally, he discovered that by holding a lighted candle near the ear, the insects would at once leave the cavity and come forth. The patient should be in the dark when this is done.

THE HEARTHSTONE, PHILADELPHIA 1883

TO EXTRACT A CLOVE, BEAN OR ANY ARTIFICIAL SUBSTANCE FROM THE NOSE OF A CHILD: Press with the finger the well nostril, so as to completely close it, at the same time fitting your lips to the child's closely, blow with a sudden puff into the child's mouth. The writer thus extracted a clove from the nose of a young child.

THE IMPROVED HOUSEWIFE, HARTFORD, 1846

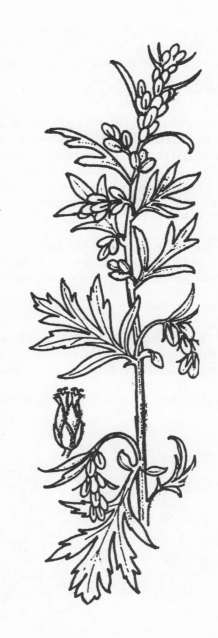

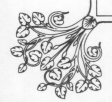
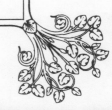

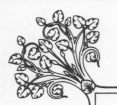

Cuts and Bleeding

'I shall desire you of more acquaintance, good Master Cobweb. If I cut my finger, I shall make bold with you.'
SHAKESPEARE, *A MIDSUMMER NIGHT'S DREAM*

BIND THE CUT with cobwebs and brown sugar, pressed on like lint: Or if you can not procure these, with the fine dust of tea.
THE HEARTHSTONE, PHILADELPHIA 1883

TO STOP BLEEDING IF THE VEINE BE CUT ASUNDER: Take the shell of goose or hen that the chick comes out of when hatched and make it into a powder being first burnt and cast thereon and it stanch it presently. . .Probatum Est.
A BOOK OF SIMPLES, C. 1750

COUNT BACKWARDS from fifty, inclusive until you come down to three. As soon as you arrive at three, you will be done bleeding.
THE LONG LOST FRIEND, 1856

WRITE THE WORD 'Veronica' with pen and ink on ye ball of ye left thumb and it will in a very short time stop ye bleeding.
A PLAIN PLANTAIN, 17TH C. HOUSEHOLD RECEIPT BOOK

IN THE FALL of the year gather puffballs when they have turned brown and are filled with a very fine dust, and put them carefully away. When needed cut open a puffball and apply the cut surface of the ball to the wound. It will stop the blood.
NORTH AMERICAN PIONEER REMEDY

North American settlers learned this remedy from the Indians who used the puff ball for several cures. As well as being applied to wounds, it was put on the umbilicus of new-born infants, used as a talcum powder to cure chafing on babies, and applied in the treatment of broken ear drums.

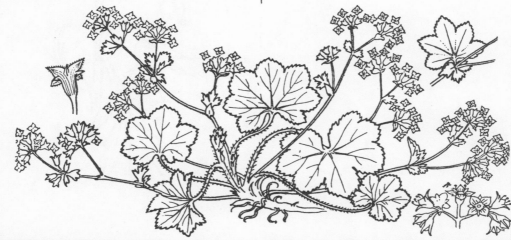

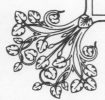
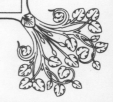

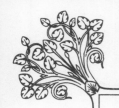

Go thou, I'll fetch some Flax and whites of eggs
To apply to his bleeding face.
SHAKESPEARE, *KING LEAR*

IF A WOUND BLEEDS very fast and there is no physician at hand, cover it with scrappings of sole leather, scrapped like coarse lint. This stops blood very soon. Always have vinegar, camphor, hartshorn, or something of that kind, in readiness, as the sudden stoppage of blood almost always makes a person faint.
LYDIA CHILD, *THE FRUGAL HOUSEWIFE*, BOSTON, 1831.

TAKE A PIECE of blue cloth and burn it in the fire and lay it to the wound and it will cease.
STERE ITT WELL

IT IS CLAIMED that bleeding may be stopped, on man or beast, by binding on a mixture of equal parts of wheat flour and salt; of course they are not to be wet, but evenly mixed before binding on. The blood does the wetting.
DR. CHASE'S RECIPES, 1867

THE LEAVES OF GERANIUM are an excellent application for cuts, where the skin is rubbed off, and other wounds of that type. One or two leaves must be bruised and applied to the part and the wound will be cicatrized in a short time.
THE FARMER'S ADVOCATE, LONDON, ONTARIO, MAY 1885

CUTS: Keep it closed with your thumb a quarter of an hour. Then double a rag five or six times, dip it in cold water and bind it on. Tried. Or bind on toasted cheese. This will cure a deep cut. Or pounded grass. Shake it off after twelve hours, and, if need be, apply fresh.
REVEREND JOHN WESLEY, *PRIMITIVE PHYSICK*, 1747

TO STOP PAINS OR SMARTING IN A WOUND: Cut three small twigs from a tree—each to be cut off in one cut. Rub one end of each twig in the wound, and then wrap them separately in a piece of white paper and put them in a warm and dry place.
THE LONG LOST FRIEND, 1856

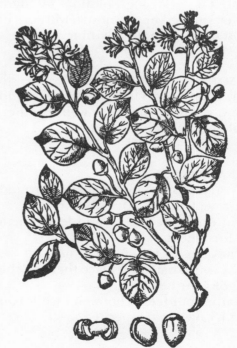

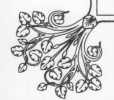
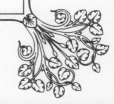

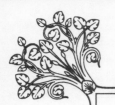

Nosebleeds

TAKE A DRIED TOAD, sew it in a bag and wear it at the pit of the stomach ...this will stop a bleeding at the nose.
THE FAMILY MAGAZINE, LONDON, 1741

PUT A LARGE KEY suddenly down the back, or a small piece of writing paper under the tongue; either will effect a cure.
THE HOUSEKEEPER'S ALMANAC, NEW YORK, 1842

A FRENCH SURGEON says that the simple elevation of a person's arm will stop the bleeding at the nose. He explains the fact physiologically and declares it a positive remedy. It is certainly easy of trial. Or, a strong solution of alum water, snuffed up the nostril will cure in most cases, without anything further.
THE HEARTHSTONE, PHILADELPHIA 1883

A SIMPLE CURE for nosebleed is to crowd the fingers tight into the ears and chew, pressing the teeth well together, as if chewing food.
DR CHASE'S RECIPES, 1892 EDITION

TEXAS REMEDIES:
• Wear a piece of pure lead tied around your neck with a pure silk thread.
• Put on clean clothes and leave them on for nine days.
• Put strips of bacon in the nose.
• Cross two nails and place them on the top of your head.
• Bathe your feet in hot water while you drink cayenne pepper tea.

TAKE THE MOSS of an ashen tree gathered on the sunny side, shred it small, mix with bole armoniack and strong white wine vinegar; make it into paste and apply it to the wrists, temples and nostrils.
A PLAIN PLANTAIN, 17TH. C.
HOUSEHOLD RECEIPT BOOK

EXTRAORDINARY AS IT MAY APPEAR, a piece of brown paper folded and placed between the upper lip and the gum, it is said will stop bleeding of the nose.
THE CANADA FARMER, TORONTO, 16 MAY, 1864

RUB YOUR NOSTRILS with the juice of nettles or round nettles, bruised.
THE FAMILY MANUAL, NEW YORK, 1845

TO STAUNCH BLOOD FALLING FROM THE NOSE BY A SIMPLE HELD IN ONE'S HAND: Let the patient hold knot-grass and solomen's seal in his hand till it grow warm there, or longer, if need be.
THE COMPLETE FAMILY PIECE AND COUNTRY GENTLEMAN AND FARMER'S BEST GUIDE, LONDON, 1741

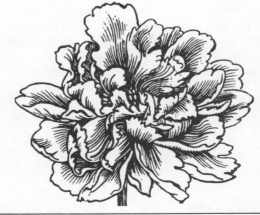

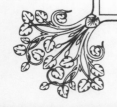

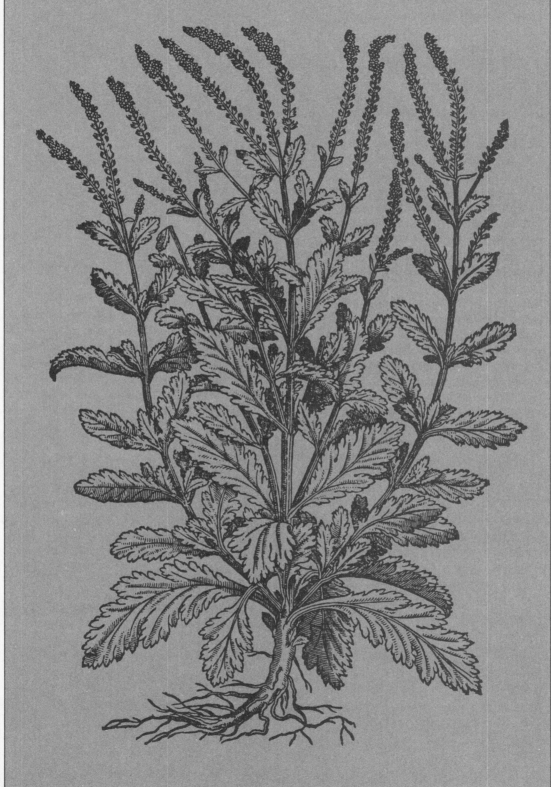

TO PREVENT NOSEBLEEDS:

Drink whey largely every morning, and eat much raisons.

Or, dissolve two scruples of nitre in half a pint of water, and take a teacupful every hour.

To cure it, apply to the neck behind and on each side, a clothe dipped in cold water.

Or, put the legs and arms in cold water.

Or, wash the temples, nose and neck with vinegar.

Or, keep a little roll of white paper under the tongue.

Or, snuff up vinegar and water.

Or, foment the legs with it.

Or, steep a linen cloth in sharp vinegar, burn it and blow it up the nose with a quill.

Or, apply tents made of soft lint dipped in cold water, strongly impregnated with tincture of iron and introduced within the nostrils quite through to their posterior apertures. This method, Mr Heys says never failed him.

In a violent case, go into a pond or river.

REVEREND JOHN WESLEY, *PRIMITIVE PHYSICK*, 1747

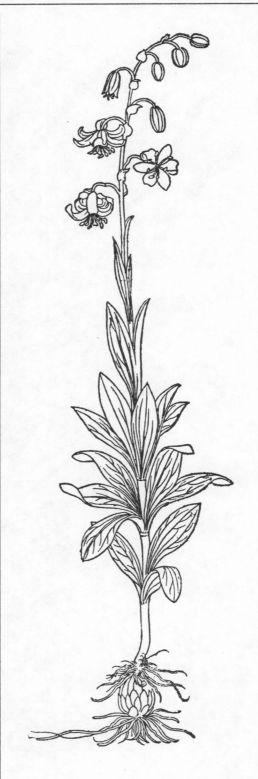

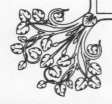

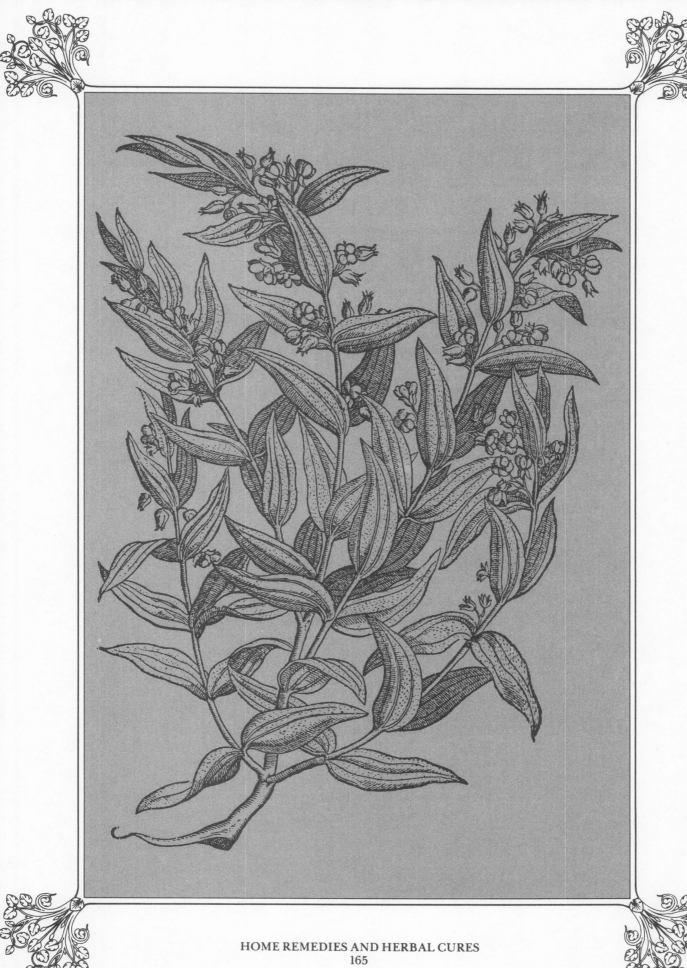

Frostbite

TAKE A WHITE WOOLEN CLOTH which has never been used before, burn it to ashes, strew these ashes upon the afflicked feet and they will heal.
ALBERTUS MAGNUS OR EGYPTIAN SECRETS

FOR FROSTED FEET OR LIMBS, take hog's lard and snow, equal parts and grease three evenings with it.
JOHN STONER'S SYMPATHY, 1867.

KENTUCKY MOUNTAIN REMEDIES:
• A remedy for frozen feet is to wrap the feet in the skins of rabbits killed in the dark of the moon.
• Bury a crooked penny at the north-east corner of the cabin outside where water drops from the eaves.
KENTUCKY SUPERSTITIONS, 1920

TEXAS REMEDIES:
• Soak feet in an ashes and water solution.
• Kill a chicken and soak the damaged feet or hands in the warm blood.
• Mix cow manure and milk, place in a cloth and apply to the frost bitten area.

TAKE HYDROCHLORIC ACID, one ounce; rain water, seven ounces; wash the feet with it two or three times daily, or wet the socks with the preparation until relieved. A gentleman whose feet had been frozen in the alps, eight years before and another man's had been frozen two years before on the Sierra Nevada mountains, were effectively cured by its use.
DR CHASE'S RECIPES, 1867 EDITION

IT IS SAID that an Indian meal poultice covered with young hyson tea, softened with hot water and laid over the burns or frozen flesh, as hot as can be borne, will relieve the pain in five minutes.
AVERY'S ALMANACK, NEW BRUNSWICK, 1857

STEEP A PIECE OF LIME for six hours and then for every two spoonfuls of water, add one of linseed oil; stir until it becomes an ointment of the substance of cream and then apply to the place affected. This is worthy of a trial.
THE CANADA FARMER, TORONTO, 1 MARCH, 1865

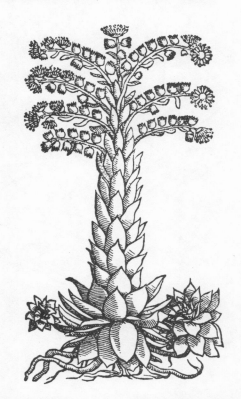

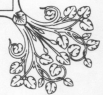

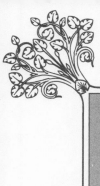
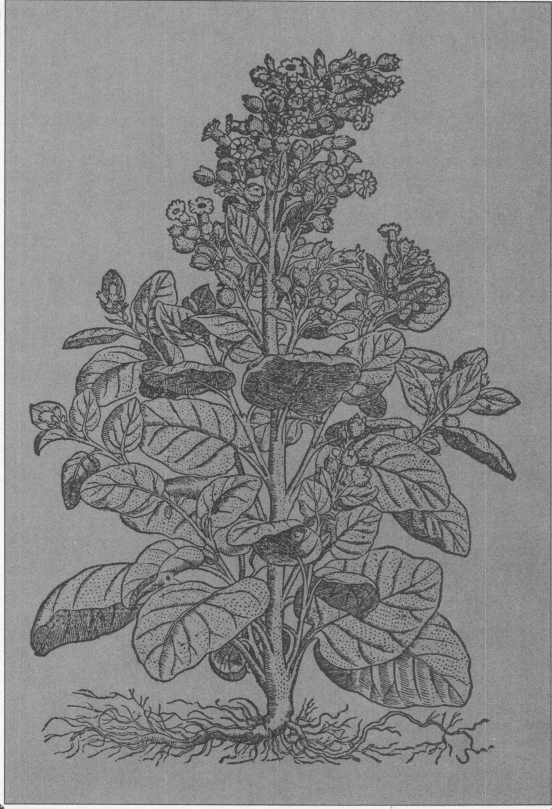

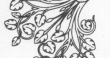

Poison Ivy

WHEN THE ERUPTION first appears, heat a flat piece of iron to redness, hold it while hot near the irritated parts until the effects of the heat are a little painful. The eruption will progress no further, and the swelling, if any, will subside.
FARMER'S DIRECTORY AND HOUSEKEEPER'S ASSISTANT, TORONTO, 1851

APPALACHIAN FOLK REMEDIES:
• Use a mixture of buttermilk or vinegar and salt.
• Make a strong brown tea by boiling willow leaves and put the tea on the affected area.
• Rub wild touch-me-not on the area.
• Rub the infection with the inside of a banana skin.

TEXAS REMEDIES:
• Rub the ashes of the huajillo root on it.
• Apply a mixture of gunpowder and cream.
• Apply boiled pecan leaves.
• Rub the milk from milkweed directly on the rash.
• Rub the infected area with fresh mud or cow dung every day until the redness clears up. It is best to wash every day as this removes the infection that has been drawn out during the day.

FOR EXTERNAL POISONING, take the leaves of the common soup bean and bruise them to a pulp: Apply to the affected parts and change every hour. The dry beans ground up and mixed with water are just as good.
THE PEOPLE'S HOME MEDICAL BOOK, CLEVELAND, OHIO, 1916

A SIMPLE AND EFFECTUAL REMEDY for ivy poisoning is said to be sweet spirits of nitre. Bathe the affected parts two or three times during the day and the next morning scarely any trace of the poison will remain.
BUCKEYE COOKERY, MINNEAPOLIS, 1881

BOIL ONE HALF PINT OF SHELLED OATS in water until the latter is really dark, and use this oat tea to wash the poisoned parts.
ONTARIO PIONEER REMEDY

BROMINE, fifteen grams; rubbed in one ounce of olive oil, or glycerine and apply three or four times daily; one application at bed-time has been found effectual; a poultice of clay-mud has also cured many cases ...
OR
Take one pint of the bark of black spotted alder and one quart of water and boil down to one pint. Wash the poisoned parts a dozen times a day, if convenient, it will not injure you.
DR CHASE'S RECIPES, 1892 EDITION

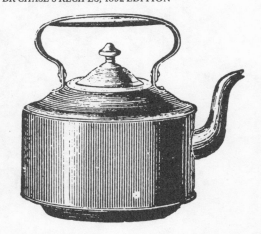

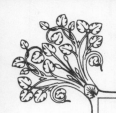

Splinters and Thorns

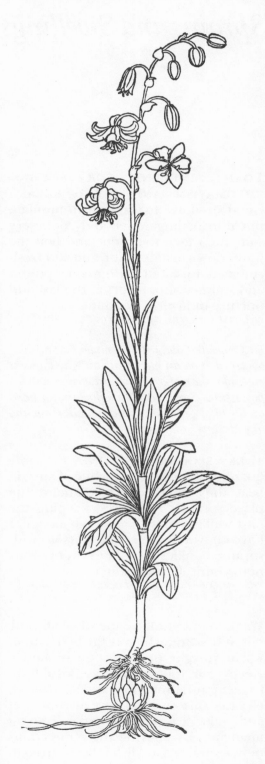

APPLY TO THEM the inner green rind of hazel, freshly scrapped.
THE HOUSEKEEPER'S ALMANAC, NEW YORK, 1842

TAKE CARROTS bruised with honey and make a powder thereof. Put over the injury, it will draw out the substance and soothe the pains.
EGYPTIAN SECRETS OR ALBERTUS MAGNUS

TAKE A LITTLE BLACK SOAP, and chew some nut-kernels, to mix with the soap and lay it on the place grieved; repeat 'till the thorn comes out.
A COLLECTION OF RECEIPTS IN COOKERY, PHYSICK AND SURGERY, LONDON, 1749

TAKE A WHITE GARLIC ONION, cut it fine, take the same weight of pitch, render the pitch down and dissolve the onions therein until it becomes the thickness of a plaster, which must be put upon the sore spot which soon heal, and the thorn may be easily removed.
ALBERTUS MAGNUS OR EGYPTIAN SECRETS

APPLY NETTLE ROOTS AND SALT. Or, turpentine spread on leather.
REVEREND JOHN WESLEY, *PRIMITIVE PHYSICK*, 1747

A Kentucky folk belief says that after you've extracted a splinter, there will be no pain if you put the splinter in your hair.

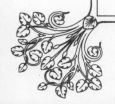
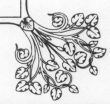

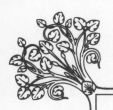

Sprains and Swellings

TOAD OINTMENT FOR SPRAINS, RHEUMATISM AND CAKED BREAST: Good sized live toads, four in number, put into boiling water and cook very soft; then take them out and boil the water down to half a pint, and add fresh churned unsalted butter, one pound and simmer altogether; at the last add tincture of arnica, two ounces.
DR CHASE'S RECIPES, 1867 EDITION

Dr Chase felt obliged to comment, 'This was obtained from an old physician who thought more of it than of any other prescription in his possession. Some people might think it hard on the toads, but you could not kill them any quicker any other way.'

TAKE A SPOONFUL OF HONEY, the same quantity of salt, and the white of an egg, beat the whole together, anoint the place sprained with this, keeping the part well rolled with a good bandage. I have known this to enable persons with sprained ankles to walk in twenty-four hours entirely free from pain.
THE FAMILY PHYSICIAN AND FARMER'S COMPANION, SYRACUSE, NEW YORK, 1840

WASH THE ANKLE frequently with cold salt and water, which is far better than warm vinegar or decoction of herbs. Keep your foot as cold as possible to prevent inflammation and sit with it elevated on a cushion. Live on a low diet and take every day some cooling medicine. By obeying these directions only, a sprained ankle has been cured in a few days.
THE FAMILY MANUAL, NEW YORK, 1845.

TAKE OF SPIRITS OF TURPENTINE, proof brandy, neats-foot oil, urine and beef's gall, each one glass, adding one teaspoonful of fine salt; mix and simmer them together, and rub on the affected parts as hot as can be borne; or take one ounce of ginger, the whites of two eggs, and one teaspoonful of fine salt; make them into a poultice and lay it on the parts affected.
LADIES INDISPENSABLE ASSISTANT, NEW YORK 1851

SWELLINGS: Nothing is so good to take down swellings, as a soft poultice of stewed white beans, put into a thin muslin bag, and renewed every hour or two.
LYDIA CHILD, *THE FRUGAL HOUSEWIFE*, BOSTON, 1831

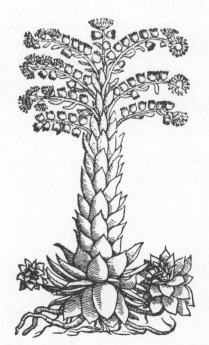

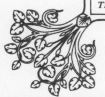
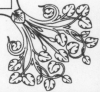

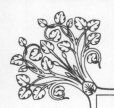

Stings

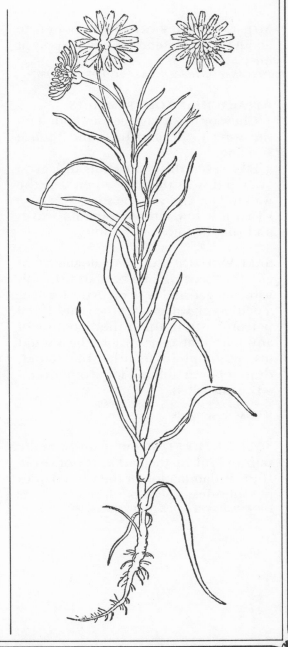

A VENOMOUS STING: Apply the juice of honey-suckle leaves.

Or, apply a poultice of bruised plantain and honey.

Or, take inwardly, one drachm of black currant leaves, powdered. It is an excellent counter-poison.

REVEREND JOHN WESLEY, *PRIMITIVE PHYSICK*, 1747.

TO TAKE THE POYSON OUT OF ANY PLACE THAT IS STUNG BY A VENEMOUS CREATURE: Hold the place upwards, for it is the manner of poysons to run upwards, if your hand be stung and you hold it down it runs up to your shoulder. Then get young pigeons and hold them to your place till they dy in your hand and so take another and another until you can see no more will dy.

CURIOUS OLD COOKERY RECEIPTS INCLUDING SIMPLES FOR SIMPLE AILMENTS, LONDON, 1891

NETTLE STING: Can be cured by rubbing the part with rosemary, mint or sage leaves.

DR CHASE'S RECIPES, 1880 EDITION

IT IS USUAL to rub the place stung with a dock leaf and say —
Nettle out, dock in,
Dock remove the nettle sting.
OLD ENGLISH CHARM CURE

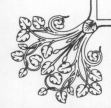

Bee Sting

Full merrily the humble-bee doth sing,
Till he hath lost his honey and his sting;
And being once subdued in armed tail,
Sweet honey and sweet notes together fail.
SHAKESPEARE, *TROILUS AND CRESSIDA*

MIX COMMON EARTH with water to about the consistency of mud. Apply at once.
THE CANADIAN HOME COOK BOOK, TORONTO, 1877

APPALACHIAN FOLK REMEDIES:
• Chew or mash ragweed and put it on the sting to deaden pain and reduce swelling.
• Take seven different kinds of leaves. Wad and twist them together, tear the wad in half and rub the sting.
• Crush a few chrysanthemum leaves and rub the juice on the sting.

SALT AND VINEGAR is a valuable remedy for the sting of a bee. Wet the salt with vinegar, and lay it on in the form of a poultice; it will extract the virus. If the person is stung upon the hand, or in any part that is accessible, he should instantly apply his mouth to the wound, draw it powerfully, till some other remedy is provided.
THE PEOPLE'S MANUAL, WORCESTER, MASSACHUSETTS, 1848

SQUEEZE THE STING out if any be in the skin and rub on the part a little olive oil. If the inflammation of the wound does not subside, apply a poultice.
THE EMIGRANT'S GUIDE TO AUSTRALIA, 1853

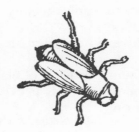

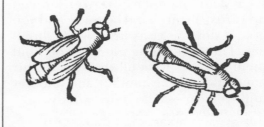

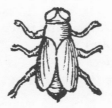

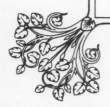
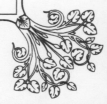

Wasp Sting

Of all the plagues that Heaven has sent, A wasp is most impertinent.
JOHN GRAY, *FABLES*, 1727

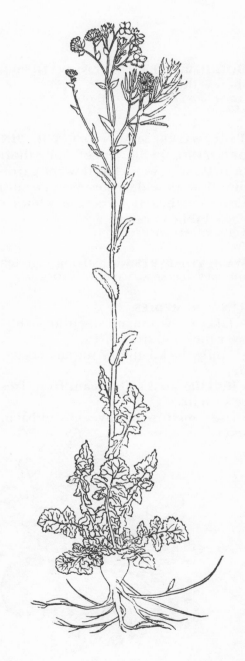

TAKE THREE KINDS of vegetables, pound them together and squeeze out the juice; apply this, and it will seldom fail to give speedy relief.
THE FAMILY PHYSICIAN AND FARMER'S COMPANION, SYRACUSE, NEW YORK, 1840

PRESS THE PIPE of a key upon the part stung for a minute or two when the pain will cease and the swelling disappear.
THE HOUSEKEEPER'S ALMANAC, NEW YORK, 1842

A LIVERPOOL PAPER STATES AS FOLLOWS: A few days ago, happening to be in the country, we witnessed the efficacy of the remedy for the sting of a wasp mentioned in one of our late papers. A little boy was stung severely and was in great torture, until an onion was applied to the part affected, when the cure was instantaneous. This important and simple remedy cannot be too generously known and we pledge ourselves to the fact above stated.
THE LONG LOST FRIEND, 1856

SIMPLE AND EFFECTUAL CURE FOR THOSE WHO MAY ACCIDENTLY HAVE SWALLOWED A WASP: Instantly, on the alarming accident taking place, put a teaspoonful of common salt in your mouth, which will instantaneously not only kill the wasp, but at the same time heal the sting.
NEW FAMILY RECEIPT BOOK, LONDON, 1815

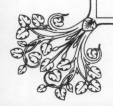
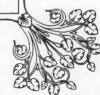

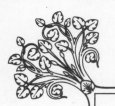

Sunburn and Sunstroke

BOIL IN BUTTER tender ivy twigs, smear therewith.
LEECH BOOK OF BALD, EARLY ANGLO-SAXON REMEDY

TAKE WATER DRAWN OFF THE VINE DROPPING, the flowers of white thorn, bean flowers, water lilly flowers, garden lilly flowers, elder flowers and tansie flowers, athea flowers, the whites of eggs, French brandy.
A QUEEN'S DELIGHT, 1671

WASH THE PARTS with strong sage tea.
THE HOUSEKEEPER'S ALMANAC, NEW YORK, 1842

TEXAS REMEDIES:
• Take a raw tomato open and rub it over the sunburned area.
• Apply thick laundry starch and let it dry.
• Rub the area with cream from fresh cow's milk.
• Use a mixture of olive oil and baking soda.

BUTTERMILK AND BRAN TEA: Wash the face before retiring with buttermilk and in the morning wash with a weak bran tea with a little cologne added.

Strawberries: Rub crushed strawberries over the face at night, writes a lady who has tried it.

Elderflower tea and cologne: Put a few drops of cologne into some elder flower tea and bathe the face for sunburn.

Cucumbers: Slice some cucumbers and let them stand in water for some time. Wash the face and hands in this water.
THE PEOPLE'S MEDICAL BOOK, CLEVELAND, OHIO, 1916

SUNTAN LOTION: That all the body may be of a clean and glad and bright hue, take oil and dregs of old wine equally much, put them into a mortar, mingle well together, and smear the body with this in the sun.
LEECH BOOK OF BALD, EARLY ANGLO-SAXON REMEDY

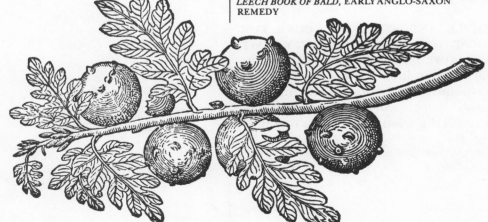

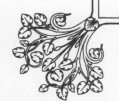
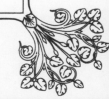

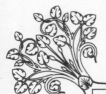
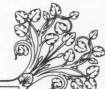

SUNSTROKE: Immediately bruise horse-radish and apply it to the stomach and give him gin to drink. Never failing.
SIX HUNDRED RECEIPTS WORTH THEIR WEIGHT IN GOLD, PHILADELPHIA, 1890

ESSENCE OF GINGER: Put the patient in a sitting position and pour cold water freely upon the head. Into half a tumbler of water pour two or three teaspoonfuls of essence of ginger and have the patients drink it quickly.
THE PEOPLE'S HOME MEDICAL BOOK, CLEVELAND, OHIO, 1916

TO PREVENT SUNSTROKE: Wear a cool cabbage leaf inside the crown of the hat. This sounds very simple but it is worth remembering.
THE AUSTRALIAN HOUSEHOLD MANUAL, 1899

PRICKLY HEAT: Keep the body gently open and rub it well with parsley.
THE HOUSEKEEPER'S ALMANAC, NEW YORK, 1842

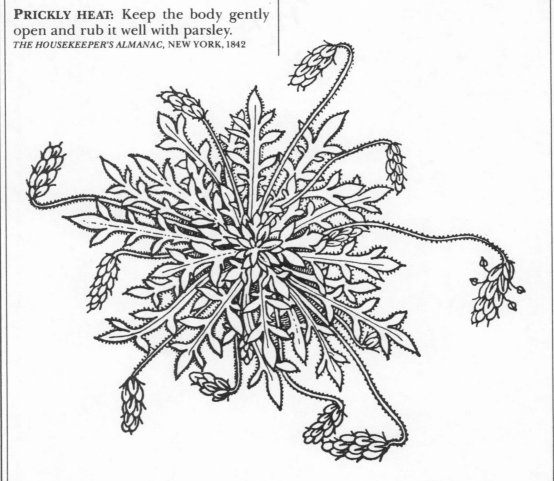

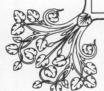
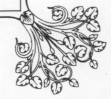

CHAPTER FIVE

Household Tips

Most of the old home-remedy books contained a random assortment of medical recipes, cookery and household tips, animal husbandry and horticultural advice. A recipe for tomato ketchup could be followed by a description of how to deworm a horse. Often the newspapers and magazines had a column devoted to friendly advice for the homemaker. And without our modern appliances, synthetic and easy-to-care-for fabrics, disposable or unbreakable containers, convenience foods and all the service industries, she needed all the help she could get. A wife or mother was busy every minute of the day, not only caring for her family and cooking over a fire or wood-burning stove, but also making her own soaps and toiletry products, reviving yellowing lace, washing kid gloves, repairing or waterproofing boots, mending broken dishes, making inks and dyes, and gathering and preserving herbs and plants for the medicines. Since most of the advice in these old books is outdated, I have only included some of the tips which might still be useful today if you want to try and save a little money or be more self-reliant. There are also tips for a more successful life. After all, where else can you find out how to deal with gossips, chatterers and scandal mongers today?

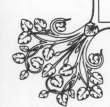

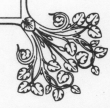

CARE OF A COFFEE POT: A carelessly kept coffee pot will impart a rank flavour to the strongest infusion of the best Java. Wash the coffee pot throughly every day and twice a week boil borax in it for fifteen minutes.
FARMER'S AND HOUSEKEEPER'S CYCLOPAEDIA, NEW YORK, 1888

TO KNOW WHETHER A BED BE DAMP OR NOT: After the bed is warmed, put a glass goblet in between the sheets and if the bed be damp, in a few minutes, drops of wet will appear in the inside of the glass. This is of great consequence to be attended to in travelling, as many have laid the foundation of incurable disorders by sleeping in a damp bed.
THE HOUSEHOLD BOOK OF PRACTICAL RECEIPTS, LONDON, 1871

TO TAKE MILDEW OUT OF LINEN: Take soap and rub it well; then scrape some fine chalk and rub that also in the linen; lay it on the grass; as it dries wet it a little and it will come out at twice.
U.S. PRACTICAL RECEIPT BOOK, 1844

HOW TO CUT GLASS: It is not generally known that glass may be cut under water with a strong pair of scissors. If a round or oval be required, take a piece of common window glass, draw the shape upon it in a black line, sink it with your left hand under water as deep as you can without interferring with the view of the line, and with your right, use the scissors to cut away what is not required.
FARMER'S AND HOUSEKEEPER'S CYCLOPAEDIA, NEW YORK, 1888

TO CLEAN GOLD AND RESTORE ITS LUSTRE: Dissolve a little sal-ammoniac in urine, boil your solid gold therein, and it will become clean and brilliant.
NEW FAMILY RECEIPT BOOK, LONDON, 1815

TO SHARPEN SCISSORS: Take a coarse sewing needle and hold it firmly between the thumb and forefinger of the left hand; then take the scissors in your right hand and cut them quickly and smoothly from hand to point. The dullest scissors, unless they are entirely worn out, can soon be sharpened in this way.
FARMER'S AND HOUSEKEEPER'S CYCLOPAEDIA, NEW YORK, 1888

TO TAKE STAINS OF WINE OUT OF LINEN: Hold the articles in milk that is boiling on the fire and the stains will soon disappear.
THE HOUSEHOLD BOOK OF PRACTICAL RECEIPTS, LONDON, 1871

TO GET RID OF THE SMELL OF OIL PAINT: Plunge a handful of hay into a pail full of water and let it stand in the room newly painted.
THE HOUSEHOLD BOOK OF PRACTICAL RECEIPTS, LONDON, 1871

TO REMOVE TAR: Rub well with clean lard, afterwards with soap and warm water. Apply this to either hands or clothing.
THE HOME COOK BOOK, TORONTO, 1884

TO PREVENT THE FORMATION OF A CRUST IN THE BOTTOM OF YOUR KETTLE: Keep an oyster shell in your tea kettle. By attracting the strong particles to itself, it will prevent the formation of a crust.
THE FAMILY MANUAL, NEW YORK, 1845

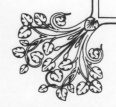

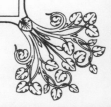

TO GET RID OF FLEAS: Leaves of the common Alder Tree —the said leaves gathered while the morning dew is on them, and brought into a chamber troubled with fleas will gather them thereunto, which being suddenly cast out will rid the chamber of those troublesome bedfellows.
NICHOLAS CULPEPER, THE ENGLISH PHYSICIAN, 1652

AN EXCELLENT FLEA TRAP: If you should happen to have the consciousness of having a flea about your person, you have but to introduce a piece of new flannel between the sheets, on placing yourself there, and you may depend on finding yourself forsaken for the flannel.
THE HOUSEHOLD BOOK OF PRACTICAL RECEIPTS, LONDON, 1871

REMEDY AGAINST FLEAS: Fumigation with brimstone or the fresh leaves of pennyroyal sewed in a bag, and laid in the bed will have the desired effect.
NEW FAMILY RECEIPT BOOK, LONDON, 1815

DOGS AND CATS: Fleas and vermin on dogs may be destroyed by bathing them in a strong infusion of lobelia for two or three mornings, washing with soap and water after each application.
A NEW ENGLAND REMEDY

TO KILL COCKROACHES: A teacup full of well bruised plaster of paris, mixed with double the amount of oatmeal, to which a little sugar (the latter is not essential) then strew it on the floor or in the chinks where they frequent.
THE HOUSEHOLD BOOK OF PRACTICAL RECEIPTS, LONDON, 1871

TO DESTROY ANTS: Put red pepper in the places ants frequent the most and scrub the shelves and drawers with strong carbolic soap.
Red ants may be banished from a pantry or storeroom by strewing the shelves with a small quantity of cloves, either whole or ground. The cloves should be renewed occasionally as after a time they lose their strength and decay.
FARMER'S AND HOUSEKEEPER'S CYCLOPAEDIA, NEW YORK, 1888

ANTS: A small quantity of green sage placed in the closet will cause red ants to disappear.
U.S. PRACTICAL RECEIPT BOOK, 1844

FLIES ON PICTURES: The following simple way of preventing flies to sit on pictures or any other furniture is well experienced and will, if generally used, prevent trouble and damage. Let a large bunch of leeks soak for four to five days in a pail of water and wash the picture or any piece of furniture with it, the flies will never come near anything so washed.
GODEY'S MAGAZINE

HOW TO DRIVE AWAY BED BUGS: Fern leaves, gathered between the last two days of the month of June, and put under the bed will drive away bed bugs sure.
ALBERTUS MAGNUS OR EGYPTIAN SECRETS

TO PRESERVE FURS FROM MOTHS ETC: Wrap up a few cloves or peppercorns with them when you put them away for any length of time, and always keep them in a dry place.
U.S. PRACTICAL RECEIPT BOOK, 1844

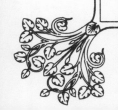
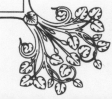

TO KEEP MOTHS, BEETLES ETC FROM CLOTHES: Put a piece of camphor in a linen bag or some aromatic herbs, in the drawers, among linen or woolen clothes and neither moth nor worm will come near them.
THE HOUSEHOLD BOOK OF PRACTICAL RECEIPTS, LONDON, 1871

A CERTAIN ART TO KILL FLIES: Take sweet milk, add black pepper to it, mix well, and leave it for the flies to eat. All flies that partake of it will die.
ALBERTUS MAGNUS OR EGYPTIAN SECRETS

TO RESTORE FROZEN PLANTS: As soon as discovered, pour cold water over the plant, wetting every leaf throughly. In a few moments it will be crystallized with a thick coating of ice. In this state place it in the dark, carefully covered with a newspaper. The ice will slowly melt, leaving the plant in its original state of health.
THE HOME COOK BOOK, TORONTO, 1884

TO EXPAND TULIPS AND OTHER FLOWERS: Tulips, and other flowers, when cut early on a dull, cold morning, are seldom very well expanded. If they are afterwards placed in a warm room and their stems put to stand in warm water, it will cause them to expand their flowers as well as they would have done on a bed in the brightest day of spring. This is not only applicable to tulips, but to many other flowers as well.
THE HOUSEHOLD BOOK OF PRACTICAL RECEIPTS, LONDON, 1871

TO PRESERVE THE NATURAL COLOR IN PETALS OF DRIED FLOWERS: Nothing more is necessary than to immerse the petals for some minutes in alcohol. The colors will fade at first; but then in a short time they will resume their natural tint and remain permanently fixed.
NEW FAMILY RECEIPT BOOK, LONDON, 1815

TO PRESERVE BARKS: Barks may be conveniently preserved, by placing them in coarse brown paper bags and hanging them up, in some airy and dry situation, until all extraneous moisture has evaporated.
U.S. PRACTICAL RECEIPT BOOK, 1844

TO GATHER AND PRESERVE HERBS: Herbs should be gathered early in a morning at the season when they are just beginning to flower. The dust should be washed or brushed off them and they should be dried by a gentle heat as quick as possible.
U.S. PRACTICAL RECEIPT BOOK, 1844

TO RESTORE FADED FLOWERS: Put the flowers into scalding hot water sufficiently high to cover one-third of their stems; let them stand until the water is cold, then cut off the soft part of the stems and place them in cold water.
U.S. PRACTICAL RECEIPT BOOK, 1844

A SURE WAY OF CATCHING FISH: Take rose seed and mustard seed and the foot of a weasel and hang these in a net and the fish will certainly collect there.
THE LONG LOST FRIEND, 1856

TO MAKE CHICKENS LAY MANY EGGS: Take the dung of rabbits, pound it to a powder, mix it with bran, wet the mixture until it forms lumps and feed your chickens with it and they will keep on laying a great many eggs.
THE LONG LOST FRIEND, 1856

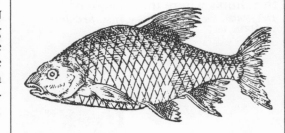

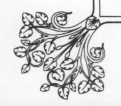
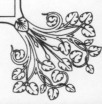

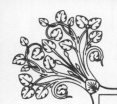

Tips for a More Successful Life

AGAINST A WOMAN'S CHATTER: Against a woman's chatter, taste at night fasting a root of radish, that day the chatter can not harm thee.
THE LEECH BOOK OF BALD, 10TH C. ANGLO-SAXON REMEDY

CURE FOR SCANDAL: Take of good nature, one ounce, of a herb commonly called by the Indians "mind your own business", one ounce, mix this with a little charity for failings and simmer them together in a vessel called circumspection for a short time, and it will be fit for use.
Application: The symptoms are a violent itching in the tongue and the roof of the mouth, which invariably takes place when you are with a kind of animal called gossips. When you feel a turn of it coming on, take a spoonful of the above, hold it in your mouth which you will keep shut, until you are out of the way of such animals and you will find a complete cure. Should you apprehend a relapse, keep a phial about you and on feeling the slightest symptom, repeat the dose.
THE LADY'S ANNUAL REGISTER, BOSTON, 1839

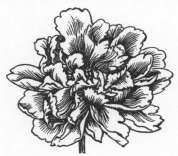

MEDICINE FOR IMPROVING THE MEMORY: Take a tablespoon full of tincture of hyssop, a single drop of oil of cinnamon. Mix and put into your last cup of tea morning and evening.
THE FAMILY ORACLE OF HEALTH, ECONOMY AND GOOD LIVING, LONDON, 1825

The Family Oracle *commented on the reasons for memory loss. 'At the very head of the causes which tend to impair and destroy the memory we place sexual indulgence.' It continued to say that it was also caused by 'all sorts of irregular living, late hours and debauchery.'*

TO WIN EVERY GAME ONE ENGAGES IN: Tie the heart of a bat with a red silken string to the right arm and you will win every game at cards you play.
THE LONG LOST FRIEND, 1856

QUARRELLING: Take a small handful of sassafras roots, place in a pint bottle, fill the bottle with water and let it stand. When anyone comes in and begins to scold you, fill your mouth with this and hold it till he goes out. A cure is guaranteed.
INGLENOOK DOCTOR BOOK, 1911

HOW TO OBTAIN THINGS WHICH ARE DESIRED: If you call upon another to ask for a favour, take care to carry a little of the fivefinger grass (cinquefoil) with you and you shall certainly obtain that you desired.
THE LONG LOST FRIEND, 1856

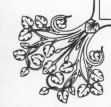
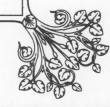

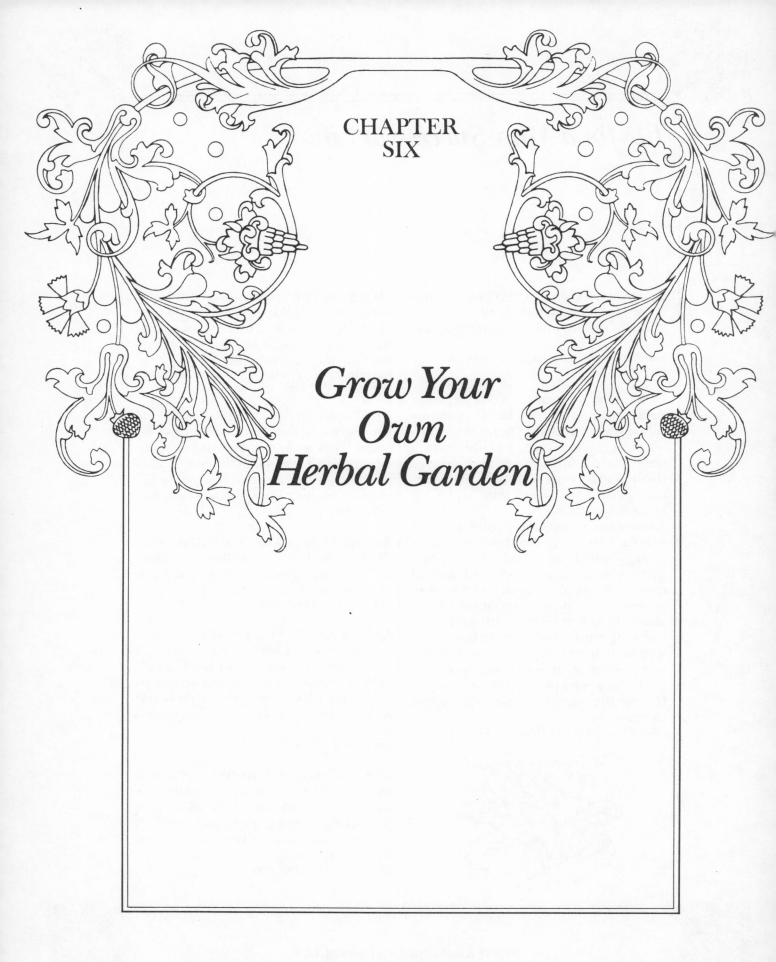

CHAPTER
SIX

*Grow Your
Own
Herbal Garden*

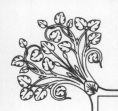

As overstated as some of the claims for 'cures' from herbal remedies might be in the old receipts books, many plants do indeed help the body heal itself. Comfrey (Symphytum officinale) has long been used as a healing agent for broken bones and damaged tissues. Scientific analysis has found that comfrey contains allantoin, a cell proliferant and 'modern' miracle healing agent. And many herbs just contain healthy amounts of vitamins and minerals which help the body's own defense mechanisms. Besides allantoin, comfrey tea contains a high dose of calcium, and vitamins A and B. Some pleasant-tasting herbs such as mint also aid in the digestion of foods, which is why the use of herbs in cooking has continued even as stronger and more bitter-tasting medicinal herbs have been relegated to the status of 'weeds'.

But the culinary herbs have not lost their old powers. Besides perking up casseroles, parsley will aid in their digestion and give you a good dose of vitamins A and C. Peter Rabbit knew what he was doing when he went to look for some parsley after eating too many of Mr. McGregor's lettuces, French beans and radishes. (And well he should — old Mrs. Rabbit sold herbs for a living.)

If you want to experiment with herbal home remedies, the delightful herbs discussed in this chapter can be grown inside your own home. If you are disappointed in the remedy you can always use them for stew.

Many of these herbs can be purchased at the grocery store but they are dried and usually expensive. Drying removes some of the volatile oils and most of the vitamins. Also, even if herbs are kept in sealed bottles, their flavour deteriorates with long storage. If you grow your own you always have fresh herbs on hand, and besides being useful, herbs make beautiful plants.

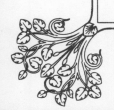
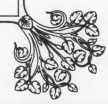

Before You Start—General Hints

Buy seeds from a good, reputable dealer. Unless the store or nursery sells a lot of them, they may not be fresh, and old seeds may not germinate at all. Herb specialists also publish helpful and fascinating seed catalogues.

Instead of sowing the seeds directly into the pot, try starting the seeds in pellets (which are sold under several trade names). When soaked in water, the pellets expand and the seeds can be planted into their mixture of peat moss and other materials. After two or three pairs of true leaves appear, the seedlings are established (the first two leaves to appear are seed leaves, not true leaves), and the pellets can be placed directly into the planting soil in the pots. While the seeds are germinating, make sure the pellets do not dry out. Set them on sand or gravel in a tray with water.

To aid germination, cover the pellets or pots with a sheet of clear plastic in which you have punched a few holes. Do not leave the plastic on all the time; remove it at night or you might just grow moulds. Watering the seedlings occasionally with camomile tea is said to prevent them from "damping off" or rotting.

Most herbs prefer a light soil. Try a mixture of one-third each potting soil, sand, and a soil substitute such as peat moss. For plants requiring a more alkaline soil, add a handful of pulverized limestone. Gravel or broken crockery should be placed in the bottom of the pot to allow proper drainage.

To increase the humidity near the plants (they hate hot, dry air), fill a metal tray with water and place it under them.

Use a high-nitrogen commercial fertilizer. Every six months, water and then rewater the plants to wash out accumulated deposits.

Tall, sparse growth is an indication that plants are not getting enough light. If you have few windows which receive sunlight for at least six hours a day, try using lights which simulate sunlight.

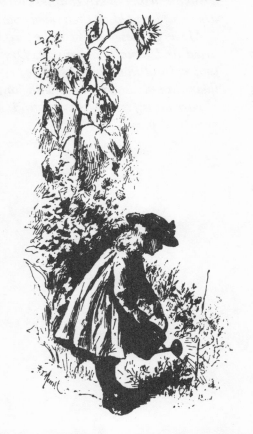

Basil

Traditionally, a pot of basil has been grown in the house to repel flies. A dwarf variety *(Ocimum minimum)* with 1 cm (½-inch) leaves is available which makes a nice, compact house plant. An annual, basil germinates easily and quickly in four to five days, so grow it from seed in a small pot. This plant loves sun and should be placed in your sunniest window. Pinch the centre stem and allow the sides to grow bushy. Remember that both the leaves and the roots of this plant require moisture.

Basil was an ingredient in snuff, as it was reputed to clear the head. Similarly, basil oil was rubbed on the temples to alleviate headaches.

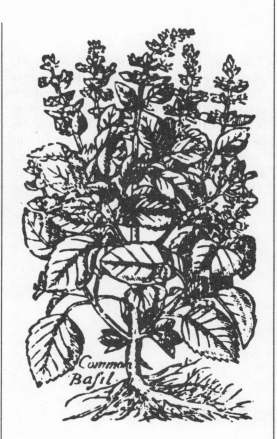

Common Basil

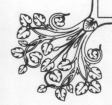
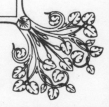

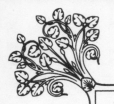

Chervil

The amateur gardener will love this plant—it grows more easily indoors than in the garden. Chervil, which tastes like a mild parsley, actually prefers shade to bright sun. This annual is easily germinated and the seeds should be sown directly in the pot as the roots are weak and best not transplanted. The leaves are said to bring relief to bruises.

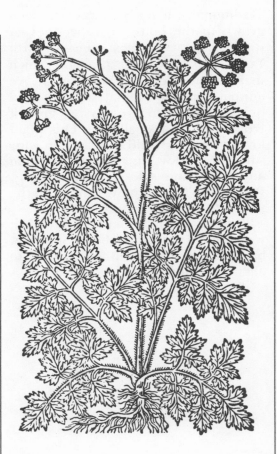

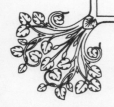
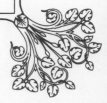

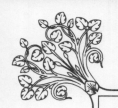

Dill

Easily grown from seed, four of these tall, feathery foliaged plants will grow in a 25-cm (10-inch) pot. Use half loam and half sand for the soil mixture and give the plant a sunny spot. It is an annual.

Dill seeds are known to be helpful in digestion; they are also contain potassium, phosphorus, sodium and sulphur.

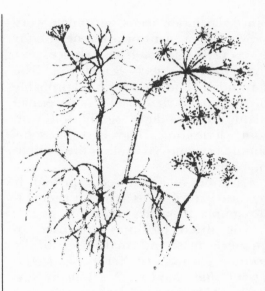

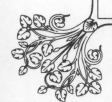
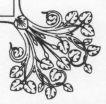

Lavender

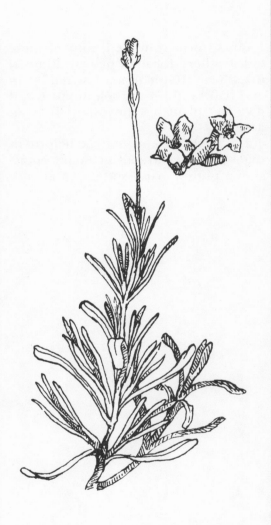

Since, lavender seeds germinate very slowly, buy a plant or ask a neighbour for a cutting. If you have a choice, selct the hardiest variety—English or True Lavender. (The French would probably dispute this claim.) This perennial plant requires light sandy soil with some limestone. The first blossoms should be removed to allow the plant to fill out.

Lavender oil is an insect repellent. It has also been used as a rub for rheumatic complaints, aches and pains.

The dried blossoms are used to enhance teas and make beautifully scented sachets. In her book, *Herbs: Their Culture and Uses* (Macmillan, New York, 1974) Rosetta Clarkson tells how to make a sachet which will prevent moths from damaging clothes:

TWO HANDFULS EACH dried lavender flowers, rosemary; one tablespoon each crushed cloves and small pieces of lemon peel.

The mixture is put into a small pad or bag.

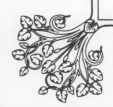
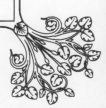

Lemon Balm

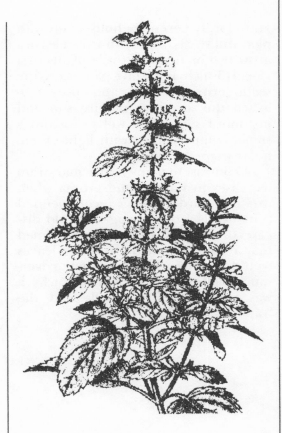

The botanical name for this fragrant plant is *Melissa officinalis. Officinalis* indicated that the herb was medicinal, 'from the apothecary shop.' The physicians of Arabia esteemed it for its healing, soothing and calming properties. Scholars drank it before examinations in order to sharpen their memories and understanding. The ancients held it to be a heart and blood restorative. In any case, a cup of lemon balm is delicious, and definitely soothing.

While this hardy perennial can be grown from seed in the spring, germination can be tricky. Soak the seeds overnight in warm water before planting. At other times of the year buy a plant. It will require light sandy soil, which should be kept a bit on the dry side. The pot should be placed in a partly shaded location.

Marjoram

For a lovely perennial houseplant with plentiful swirls of greyish-green leaves, grow two or three of these plants in a 13-cm (5-inch) pot. Have patience as the seeds germinate slowly, and once established the seedlings require sun and just-moist soil. They will grow into a small, compact bush with light-green, heart-shaped leaves.

In contrast to many herbs, marjoram increases in flavour and aroma when dried. Gerard's *Herball* recommended it highly as a remedy against cold diseases of the brain and head and claimed that a decoction made from the leaves would 'easeth such as are given to over-much sighing.' Perhaps that is why it was used for dizzy spells and the 'vapours.'

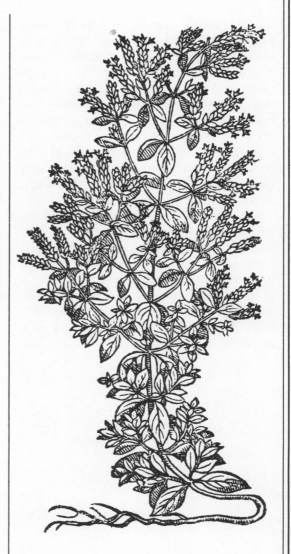

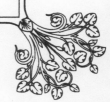

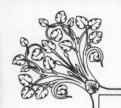

Mint

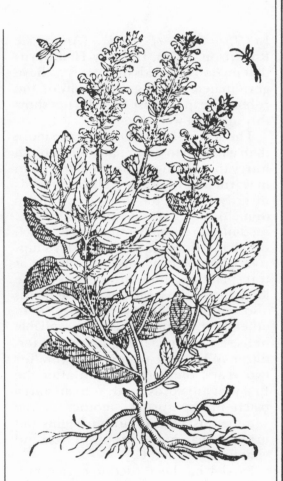

As the natural habitat of this plant is wet meadows and alongside brooks, give it rich, moist soil, plenty of sun and it will flourish. There are many varieties, but try peppermint, *Mentha piperita,* for your indoor garden. It produces the strongest aromatic oils. Buy a plant, give it a large pot and watch this perennial spread. However, the plants should always be cut back before the flowers go to seed.

Peppermint infusions have been used to aid digestion, relieve nausea, calm colicky infants and soothe the pain of headaches. The oil brings warmth wherever rubbed on the skin and some people inhale the oil to clear a stuffed nose. In any case, a cup of mint tea with lemon and honey is the best-tasting medicine you could ask for.

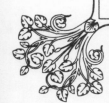
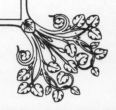

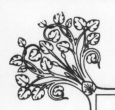

Parsley

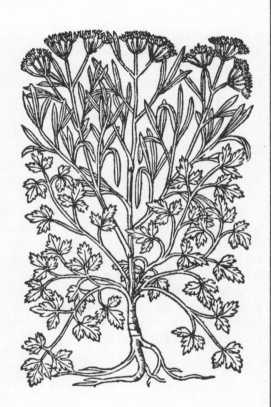

In *The Book of Herbs* (Angus & Robertson, 1972), Dorothy Hall warns that millions of seeds of parsley . . . have germinated in the garbage bin or the rubbish heap because they did not show through in a week.'

The seeds of this herb can take more than a month to germinate, but you can hurry them along by first soaking them in warm water for a day. Plant the seeds directly, but not too deeply, in a 20-cm (8-inch) pot. When those stubborn seedlings are finally established, pinch off all but three of them. Parsley's taproot will protect against any attempt at transplanting, and also grows quite long, hence the large pot. These plants also require a slightly richer soil than other herbs. Add compost if available or use a commercial, high-nitrogen fertilizer. While the plants will grow for two years, the leaves grown after the first year are not as good. You can start a batch in the spring, another in the summer just before autumn begins and insure a year-round supply of iron and vitamins A, B and C.

Parsley has been used to cure everything from baldness to rheumatism. Indeed, many generations of older people have maintained that a daily glass of homemade parsley wine will keep both body and mind young.

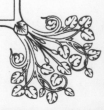

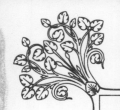

Rosemary

While it is possible to germinate rosemary from seed, this perennial grows so slowly that unless you wish to wait a year before harvesting, you should buy a plant. Once established, the plant can grow quite large, given dry, well-drained light soil—with a touch of crushed limestone —and lots of sun. As rosemary is quite tender, make sure that it is given just enough water so the roots do not suffer, and place it in an area that is cool, but humid. Keep the plant trimmed to a maximum length of 60 cm (2 feet) in a 25-cm (10-inch) pot for a most attractive houseplant. Its narrow, gray-green leaves produce a pine-like bush, which when well-cared for will be graced with pale blue flowers.

Rosemary leaves have been used as a tea for nervous headaches, even smoked as a cure for asthma and other lung complaints. However, it is most prized as an ingredient in beauty preparations such as hair rinses and oils to condition both hair and scalp. Rosemary oil is even supposed to prevent crow's-feet around the eyes.

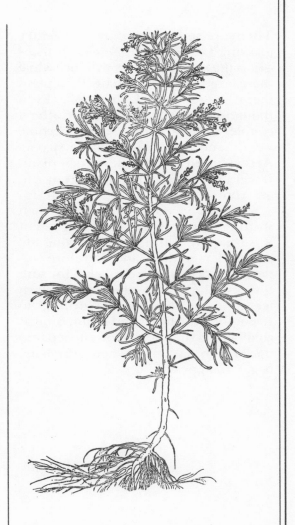

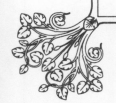
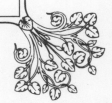

Sage

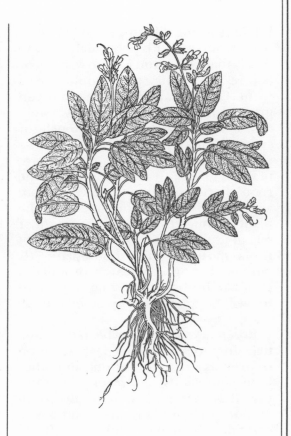

There are several varieties of sage, try growing Garden Sage, *Salvia officinalis* —it is the shortest. Have patience while these large seeds germinate, then plant them in sandy, alkaline soil. Even though sage is a perennial plant, after a couple of years the stems become woody and the oblong foliage sparse. At that time it is best to start a new plant. It will add a sharp, tingling fragrance to any room.

Sage was once valued for more than stuffing poultry—in ancient times it was believed to promote both long life and understanding, and therefore wisdom. Decoctions were gargled for sore throats, the leaves chewed to clean teeth. Sage teas were drunk to strengthen the heart and brain, combat colds—and they were even rubbed into the hair to darken it when gray hairs began to appear.

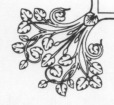
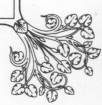

Thyme

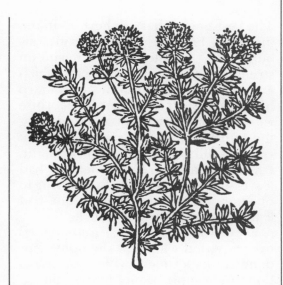

Years ago, few housewives would be without thyme in their herb gardens, because of its medicinal value. The tea was used to treat indigestion, bronchitis, whooping cough, regular coughs and many other various ailments, including melancholia in ancient Rome. Even today, wild-herb-stalker Euell Gibbons recommends thyme tea laced with honey and salt for relief of a hangover.

Thyme tea actually does kill germs. The leaves contain an essential oil, thymol, which is commercially distilled for use as an antiseptic for skin, mucus membranes and the intestinal tract, especially in the preparation of cough medicines and the treatment of hookworm and trichinosis. Large or frequent doses, however, can be poisonous.

Thyme can be easily grown from seed in the light, sandy, well-drained slightly alkaline soil that most herbs prefer. The plant also requires as much sun as possible. Of the many varieties which are available, *Thymus vulgaris* is the most popular, with its beautifully aromatic foliage and pale lavender flowers. Keep it well trimmed and this perennial will not become too woody.

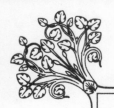

Simple Uses

The best time to harvest herbs is in the morning, because their aromatic oils build up overnight to maximum strength. Select leaves on stems which are reasonably mature, cut with a sharp implement such as a razor blade, rinse with cool or lukewarm water and hang the bunch to dry if desired, in a spot where it will not receive direct sunlight. It is important to remove dead or bad leaves and all moisture before storing in opaque, airtight containers—one bad leaf *will* spoil the whole bunch.

Even small harvests, accumulated over a period will allow the home gardener to experiment with teas, decoctions and simple beauty preparations.

TEAS. Pleasant tasting herbal teas are also called infusions or tisanes. To prepare, warm a teapot (do not use a metal one), add 15 ml (1 tablespoon) of dried herbs or a handful of fresh herbs per cup prepared and steep for ten minutes. Honey or lemon can be added to the strained tea. Tasty beverages can also be prepared by adding small amounts of herbs to ordinary tea.

DECOCTIONS. Many home remedies require decoctions, which are more concentrated than infusions, and usually more bitter. A decoction is prepared by boiling the seeds or root of the herb in water for five to ten minutes. The proportion of water to herb is usually the same as for a infusion, but can vary according to specific remedies.

BEAUTY PREPARATIONS. Two handfuls of marjoram, simmered in 227 ml or one cup of water and then rubbed lukewarm on newly washed and rinsed hair will strengthen and condition it. Or, if you have had success with your rosemary, steep a handful of that herb in a cup of boiling hot water for one hour and use instead. If possible, use soft water (rain water is ideal) for best results.

To make an herb oil, add 15 ml (1 tablespoon) of vinegar and a large handful of crushed rosemary, thyme, peppermint or lavender to a jar of safflower oil and put the lid on tight. Keep the jar in a warm place and shake the mixture once a day for a month. At the end of this time, the strained liquid is ready for use.

Fragrant rubbing lotions can be made from thyme, lavender, mint, marjoram, rosemary or lemon balm. Fill a glass jar about one-third full of your favourite herb, then add twice that amount of unscented rubbing alcohol. Let the mixture set, tightly capped, for a couple of weeks, shaking it occasionally. Strain, pour and rub away.

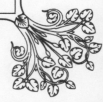

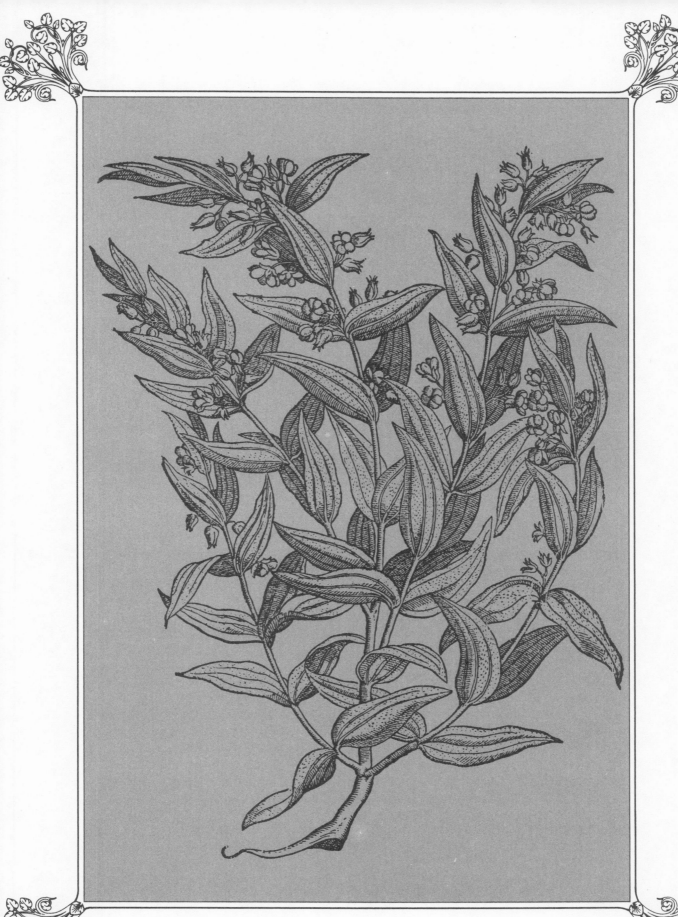

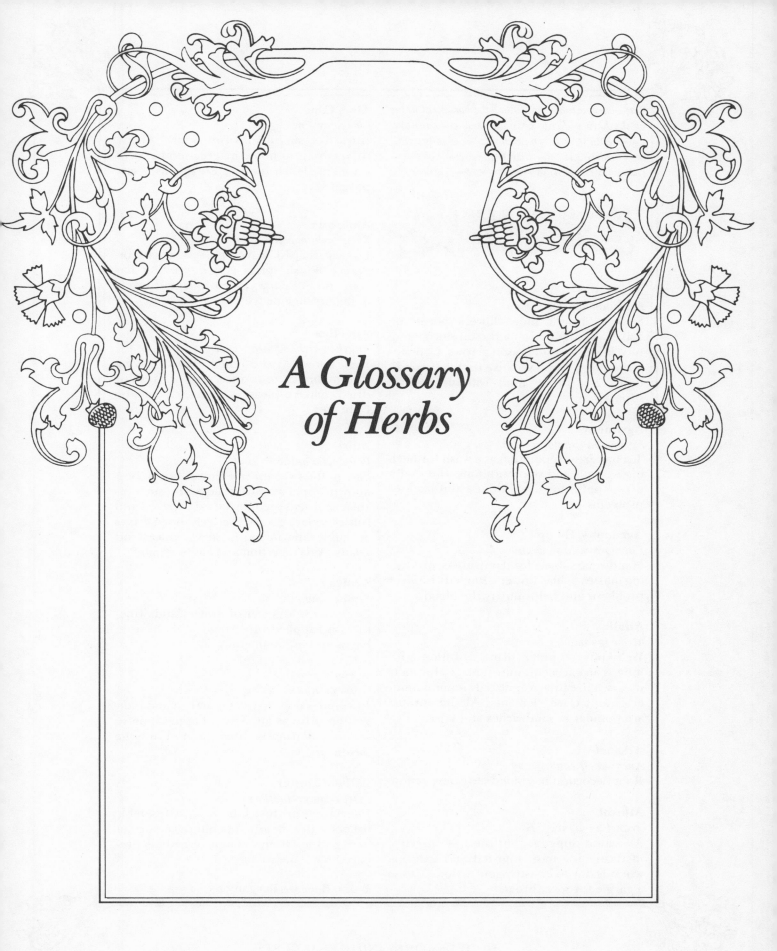

A Glossary of Herbs

The abbreviations that follow the botanical name of the herb indicate possible uses: c—culinary; d—dyeplant; h—household; i—industrial; m—medicinal; n—insecticide; p—poisonous (use with caution); s—cosmetic; t—teaplant.

Aconite
Aconitum napellus   mp
Striking bright blue flowers borne on spikes. Recognized as a poison since antiquity, it was used to poison arrows. Contains aconitine, a useful sedative for many conditions. Not to be used without medical supervision.

Agrimony
Agrimonia eupatoria   md
Tea has great reputation as a wash for healing wounds and skin eruptions. Internally, tea is useful for liver, kidney and bladder problems.

Agrimony, Hemp
Eupatorium cannabinum   m
Handsome subject for damp areas, producing masses of lilac flowers. Remedy for liver problems and helps purify the blood.

Alfalfa
Medicago sativa   cmt
Well-known fodder plant. Infusion with mint is an excellent, nutritious tea for daily use; rich in easily assimilated vitamins, minerals and trace elements. Alfalfa sprouts are popular in sandwiches and salads.

Alkanet
Anchusa officinalis   md
Root decoction has blood-cleansing action.

Allheal
Prunella vulgaris   m
As name suggests, infusion is effective medicine for most internal and external wounds due to its astringent action. Also as a gargle for sore throat.

Aloe, Cape
Aloe ferox   m
Attractive succulent from South Africa. Adapts well to home or greenhouse environment. Much used in Europe as a safe purgative.

Ambrosia
Chenopodium botrys   hm
Oakleaf-shaped leaves possess spicy fragrance. Fresh sprigs add interesting flavour to gin drinks. Dried foliage is lovely in fall arrangements.

Angelica
Angelica archangelica   cimt
Best known for candied stems, having flavour similar to licorice. Leaves, fresh or dried, make a pleasing tisane, resembling China tea.

Anise
Pimpinella anisum   cimt
One of the sweetest smelling of herbs. Best known for flavouring liqueurs such as anisette. Seeds are much used in baked and confectionary goods. Fresh chopped leaves are appealing in soups, stews, sauces and salads. Aids digestion and eases cough.

Arnica
Arnica montana   m
Protected wildflower of Switzerland. Tincture is applied externally for bruises, burns and inflammations.

Avens
Geum urbanum   m
Infusion is used to treat diarrhea and indigestion. Also as an external application to wounds. Formerly used to add unique flavour to ale.

Balloon Flower
Platycodon grandiflorus   mc
Interesting profuse blue flowers resemble balloons just before opening. Important herb of the Orient: cough remedy is prepared from the roots.

Balm, Bee. *See* Bergamot.

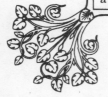

Balm, Lemon
Melissa officinalis   tcshm
The popularity of this herb is attributed to the truly delightful tea made from the dried leaves. A favourite "anytime" tea as it stimulates the heart, yet it calms the nerves. See also p. 189.

Basil. *See* p. 185

Bayberry
Myrica pensylvanica   imd
Aromatic shrub, native to the Canadian Maritimes. Astringent action of root bark abates diarrhea and hemorrhages; and as a gargle, soothes sore throat. Wax-covered berries are used to make aromatic candles and soap. Berries are boiled in water, liberating the wax, which floats on top.

Bay Laurel
Laurus nobilis   cmi
Like wine, thyme and leeks, bay leaf is a foundation flavour of French cuisine. Meat, fish and poultry dishes almost always have a touch.

Bearberry
Arctostaphylos uva-ursi   md
Creeping evergreen shrub that presents pretty waxy-looking white flowers in drooping clusters. Infusion of dried leaves in treating diseases of the bladder and kidneys is used.

Bears Breech
Acanthus mollis   m
Stately ornamental thistle featuring handsome shiny leaves of unusual shape. Decoction of leaves was once recommended for gout, burns and scalds.

Bedstraw, Yellow
Galium verum   dm
Tops and roots are sources of yellow and red dyes. Decoction is useful for bladder and kidney complaints, and has the ability to curdle milk (hence its alternate name, cheese rennet).

Belladonna
Atropa belladonna   mp
Source of atropine, valuable in treating eye diseases and spasms. External applications lessen local inflammation and pain. Should not be used without medical supervision.

Bergamot
Monarda didyma   cmit
(Bee Balm). Citrus-scented leaves and flowers make a pleasant, soothing, sleep-inducing tisane. Young leaf tips and flowers improve appearance and taste of salads. Valuable beeplant.

Betony
Stachys officinalis   mit
Good substitute for black tea; infusion resembles the taste and is caffeine-free. Helps relieve headache, and has general tonic action.

Bittersweet
Solanum dulcamara   m
Shrubby climber. Mostly used for external afflictions. Ointment made with chamomile is effective for swellings, bruises, sprains and corns. Combined with curled dock it helps skin diseases.

Borage
Borago officinalis   cmt
Known as the 'Herb of Gladness' for its exhilarating effect on the system. Add chopped young leaves and flowers to salads or summer drinks. On those sweltering summer days, cool off with iced borage tea, adding honey and lemon juice to taste.

Broom, Dyer's
Genista tinctoria   dm
Since earliest times used to dye wool bright yellow. Formerly recommended for gout and rheumatism.

Bryony
Bryonia dioica   mp
Climber. Root is a powerful purgative, rarely used for this purpose due to its drastic action. Used in homeopathy for catarrhal and rheumatic complaints. All parts are poisonous.

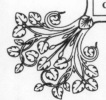

Burnet, Salad
Poterium sanguisorba cmst
Nut-cucumber flavour of leaves is welcome in salads, soups, casseroles, herb vinegars and cream cheeses. Improves the skin if added to facial treatment.

Calendula
Calendula officinalis cmst
(Pot Marigold). Flower petals give delicate flavour and strong colour to salads, omelettes and cheese, and is used as a saffron substitute for rice.

Camphor Tree
Cinnamomum camphora mi
Handsome tree from which commercial camphor is obtained. Shiny, rich green leaves are highly aromatic. Interesting pot plant for sunny window or greenhouse.

Castor Bean
Ricinus communis mpi
Oil extracted from seeds is a commonly used laxative effective for temporary constipation and acute diarrhea. Large tropical-looking foliage.

Catnip
Nepeta cataria mth
A favourite of cat lovers, for cats relish the intoxicating leaves. Tea is a popular nightcap, as it induces a good night's sleep. Valuable remedy for colds and fevers.

Catsfoot
Antennaria dioica m
Ameliorates the appetite for it stimulates bile flow, gastric juices and pancreatic secretions. Petite woolly rosettes of leaves resemble a cat's foot.

Cayenne. *See* Pepper, Cayenne.

Celandine
Chelidonium majus m
The juice mixed with vinegar is said to remove warts and corns. It was once reputed to restore eyesight. Decoction is useful for stomach pains and inflammations of the bilary duct.

Celery
Apium graveolens dulce cm
Celery juice blended with carrot and apple juice remedies poor appetite, as well as vitamin and mineral deficiency diseases.

Centaury
Centaurium erythraea m
Traditional European panacea, recommended for many complaints including lack of appetite, sluggish digestion and stomach disturbances. Highly useful during convalescence.

Chamomile
Matricaria recutita
Chamaemelum nobile mtsih
Chamomile tea, made from the flowers, is very popular in Europe as an aid to digestion, especially after heavy meals. Its soothing and cleansing effect also makes the tea a beneficial skin wash.

Chervil, Curled
Anthriscus cerefolium 'Crispum' cm
Luscious green leaves have special subtle flavour. Traditionally used in all spring soups and salads, and can improve every dish in which parsley is used. Curled leaves make a handsome garnish. See also p. 186.

Chicory, Coffee
Cichorium intybus tcm
Coffee substitute costing pennies a pound. Large roots, roasted and ground, can be blended with your favourite brand or enjoyed alone as a nourishing caffeine-free drink.

Chives
Allium schoenoprasum cm
The most delicate member of the onion family. Chopped leaves offer great improvement to salads, soups, vegetables, omelettes, and cheese dishes. Essential kitchen herb!

Cicely, Sweet
Myrrhis odorata cm
Sugar-saver. Sweet, anise-scented leaves and stalks (fresh or dried) adds delightful flavour to sweets and desserts, saving about half the sugar. Of particular interest to diabetics.

Clary
Salvia sclarea   cmi
Seeds soaked in water produce mucilaginous eye bath which safely removes particles, hence its name "clear eye" or "clary". Handsome aromatic flowers and leaves.

Clivers
Galium aparine   mhd
Fresh juice or infusion is applied to skin diseases and eruptions with good success. Said to remove freckles.

Clove-Pink
Dianthus caryophyllus   chi
Clove-scented flowers were once used to flavour ales and wines, especially celebration cups at coronations, hence its name 'carnation'. Fragrance is valuable in pot-pourris and herb sachets.

Clover, red
Trifolium pratense   m
Many herbalists assert that red clover flowers taken as an infusion help prevent and even cure cancer. Red clover is also used to treat bronchial troubles, whooping cough, gastric troubles and ulcers.

Clover Sweet. *See* Melilot.

Cohosh, Black
Cimicifuga racemosa   m
Woodland native of North America. Valued by Indians for rheumatism, kidney troubles and menstruation disorders; Indian midwives used it to relieve the pains of childbirth.

Colchicum
Colchicum autumnale   mp
(Meadow Saffron). Useful drug for gout and rheumatism, but only to be used under medical supervision. Source of colchicine, valuable to plant breeders for inducing genetic mutations. Soft lilac-pink crocus-like blooms appear in autumn.

Coltsfoot
Tussilago farfara   md
Popular remedy for respiratory conditions, including coughs, colds, hoarseness, bronchitis and bronchial asthma. Also useful in herbal smoking mixtures designed for the relief of asthma and bronchitis.

Comfrey
Symphytum officinale   mc
Comfreys are among the most important medicinal herbs. They contain allantoin, a hormone-like substance that stimulates cell division, making the comfreys valuable for healing wounds, ulcers and broken bones. Tea and poultices of leaves or roots are used. Comfreys are nutritional herbs, rich in calcium, potassium, phosphorus, vitamins and trace elements. Pound for pound they contain more protein than beefsteak. You can benefit from these nutrients by drinking the juice, or by adding finely chopped young leaves to salads. Important fodder and green manure crops as well. Can be grown indoors or out.

Coriander
Coriandrum sativum   cim
Seeds add fresh, spicy flavour to soups and stews. Main ingredient in chili sauces, curries and exotic dishes. Fresh, slightly bitter leaves, known as Chinese parsley, are featured in numerous international cuisines.

Cornflower
Centaurea cyanus   m
Striking brilliant blue blossoms, infused in water, have both curative and calming action for nervous disorders. Eyewash is reputed to strengthen weak eyes.

Cowslip
Primula veris   m
Proverbial wildflower of England, loved for its fragrant golden-yellow blossoms. Old remedy for insomnia and headache, as flowers possess sedative and nerve strengthening properties. Cowslip wine, a delicate dessert wine, has long been made from cowslip pips.

Crampbark
Viburnum opulus   mc
One of the most attractive wild shrubs. Bright red berries are used as substitute for cranberries. Cramps and spasms of all kinds succumb to bark infusions.

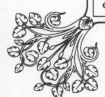

Daisy, English
Bellis perennis m
Charming button flowers appear from early spring until late autumn. Tea is employed as a gentle laxative; also for stomach and intestinal problems. Helps heal inflamed swellings and burns.

Daisy, Ox-Eye
Chrysanthemum leucanthemum m
Familiar wildflower found in meadows and along roadsides. Employed to relieve chronic cough, asthma and nervous excitability.

Dill. *See* p. 187.

Dock, Curled
Rumex crispus cmd
A valuable ointment for skin eruptions and itching is made by boiling roots in vinegar, then mixing softened pulp with lard or petroleum jelly.

Dogwood
Cornus florida mhd
Native American tree with many interesting uses. Fevers can be warded off by chewing twigs; rootbark yields a good scarlet dye; powdered bark can be made into toothpaste or a good black ink (when mixed with iron sulphate).

Dusty Miller
Senecio cineraria m
One or two drops of fresh juice dropped into the eye is said to remove cataract.

Elder
Sambucus niger cmst
Elderberries have long been used to make excellent wines and preserves. Honey-scented flowers make delightful fritters and refreshing summer drinks. Elder-flower water is commonly used in cosmetic eye and skin lotions, face packs and facial steam.

Elecampane
Inula helenium cmid
Dried root preparations quiet coughing, stimulate digestion and tone the stomach.

Epazote
Chenopodium ambrosiodes cm
(Wormseed). Strong scented foliage is highly esteemed in Mexico and Guatemala for seasoning corn, black beans, mushrooms, fish and shelfish. Wormseed oil is frequently prescribed to expel intestinal parasites.

Eucalyptus
E. globulus mih
Famous "gum" trees of Australia, sources of essential oils used in perfumery and medicine. Despite the enormous height they normally attain, they can be grown indoors with occasional pruning to maintain a manageable size. Cough drops and sore throat lozenges are made with the oil. Powerful antiseptic. Helps deodorize the air when grown indoors.

Fennel, Sweet
F. vulgare dulce cmst
Attractive lacy green foliage. Aromatic. Chopped leaves are excellent with oily fish, such as mackerel, eel and salmon, for they improve digestibility. Also used in soups, salads and stews. Fennel tea is given to infants for its calming and anti-flatulent effects.

Feverfew, Golden
Chrysanthemum parthenium 'Aureum' m
Ancient sages advised planting feverfew around homes to purify the atmosphere and ward off disease. Features decorative golden-green foliage and white daisy flowers.

Figwort
Scrophularia nodosa m
Tincture or ointment is used as a skin medication for rashes, scratches, bruises and minor wounds.

Flag, Yellow
Iris pseudacorus mchd
A beautiful plant which grows in moist shady locations. Flowers deep yellow veined with brown. Formerly employed for diarrhea and chronic cough.

Flag, Blue
Iris versicolor m
Useful for stomach, liver and gallbladder ailments. Highly regarded for migraine headache, especially when caused by stomach disorders.

Flax
Linum usitatissimum mi
Source of strong fibre used in linen cloth. Linseed poultice is valuable for rheumatism and infections. Linseed oil is employed in the paint and varnish industries.

Foxglove
Digitalis purpurea mp
Source of digitalis, important for its stimulating and regulating action on the heart, but too powerful to use without medical supervision. Spotted bells arranged in spikes are highly ornamental.

Fraxinella
Dictamnus albus m
(Gasplant). Remarkable flowers emit a gas that may be ignited on warm evenings without damage. Flowers and leaves are wonderfully fragrant of lemon when crushed.

Garlic
Allium sativum cmn
The culinary importance of garlic is only just beginning to be appreciated by North Americans. To the people of the Mediterrean, garlic conjures up such gourmet delights as escargots, Caesar salad and garlic bread. Garlic need not offend; it is often enough to rub the utensils with a clove, adding subtle flavour. Recognized medicinally, garlic capsules are sold for high blood pressure. It is also a proven antibiotic owing to its high sulphur content.

Garlic, Wild: *See* Ramsons.

Gayfeather
Liatris spicata m
Features strong spikes of deep rosy-purple flowers. Tuberous roots make a soothing tea valuable in kidney diseases or as a gargle for sore throat.

Gentian
Gentiana lutea mi
Famous European alpine herb unrivalled as a bitter tonic. Root tincture made with brandy is one of the best strengtheners of the human system, particularly in cases of weak digestion and lack of appetite.

Geranium, Scented
Pelargonium spp. chi
Available in a tantalizing array of fragrances, they have charmed window gardeners since their introduction to England in the 17th century. Leaves used in potpourris, perfumes and for flavouring preserves.

Germander
Teucrium chamaedrys m
Showy plant with glossy dark green leaves and rosy flowers. Infusion quiets upset stomach and promotes appetite. Once enjoyed considerable reputation in the treatment of gout.

Ginger, Wild
Asarum canadense cm
Woodland native of North America. Roots have ginger flavour and are much used like the popular spice. A tea made from the roots is used to relieve stomach gas.

Ginseng
Panax quinquefolius m
American ginseng is a slow-growing perennial herb found wild in cool and shady hardwood forests throughout eastern and central North America. The American ginseng root has the same properties as the Asiatic ginseng (Panax schin-seng) which has been used in the Far East for thousands of years.

The virtues of ginseng were claimed to be so fantastic that Western doctors dismissed the plant as a panacea. While these fantastic claims haven't been verified, after some 25 years of study, Russian researchers have confirmed ginseng's powerful yet harmless tonic properties. Ginseng is often prescribed by Russian doctors for those who complain of sexual failure. Also, Russian researchers found that ginseng helps build up body resistance to disease and strain, either physical or nervous.

Gipsywort
Lycopus europaeus   dm
Yields a permanent black to wool and silk. Formerly used by gypsies to darken their skin. Utilized in the treatment of palpitations of the heart.

Goats Rue
Galega officinalis   m
Handsome herb with light-blue or white flower spikes. Has supportive action in lowering blood sugar in diabetics. An extract increases lactation in cows.

Goldenrod
Solidago virgaurea   dm
Important dyeplant for its bright yellow colour. Medicinally it stimulates gastric secretions and improves the appetite. Popular Swiss herb for the expulsion of bladder stones.

Good King Henry
Chenopodium bonus-henricus   cm
Wholesome potherb. Shoots are peeled, boiled and eaten like asparagus. Young tender leaves are prepared like spinach. Excellent remedy for indigestion.

Gotu Kola
Hydrocotyle asiatica   m
Small creeping tropical plant used for centuries in India. Believed to have remarkable rejuvenating properties. One or two freshly chopped leaves daily in salads or liquified in juice are said to be sufficient to revitalize the cells of the brain and to retard the aging process. Caution must be exercised: large quantities ingested at one time have harmful narcotic effects.

Gravelroot. *See* Joe-Pye Weed.

Gumplant
Grindelia robusta   m
Efficacious for colds, coughs, nasal congestion and bronchial irritations. Also utilized as a healing wash for burns, rashes, blisters and poison ivy.

Hawthorn
Crataegus laevigata   cmh
Showy shrub with conspicuous white flowers and red berries (haws). Highly regarded as a cardiac tonic, improving blood flow in the coronary arteries and helping to regulate the heart.

Hearts-Ease
Viola tricolor   m
Old English favourite. Charming purple, lavender and yellow flowers held former romantic connotations between courting couples. Medicinally used for dropsy, respiratory catarrh and skin eruptions.

Heliotrope
Heliotropium arborescens   mi
Sweet scented violet-blue flowers are favourites as potplants or outdoor bedding plants. Cultivated for perfumery and for scenting bathing waters. Has been used for 'clergyman's sore throat.'

Hellebore, Black
Helleborus niger   mp
Cherished for its lovely white or pink-tinged blossoms. Roots are narcotic; valuable for nervous and cardiac disorders, but should only be used under medical supervision.

Hemlock, Poison
Conium maculatum   nmp
In the fresh state all parts are very poisonous. Juice was used in early times to execute criminals. Socrates died in this manner. Under proper directions it is a useful sedative for cases of nervous motor disturbances. The active principle, coniine, has proved to be an effective insecticide against aphids and blowflies.

Henbane
Hyoscyamus niger   mp
Powerful cerebral and spinal sedative used since remote ages to induce sleep and allay pains. Often an ingredient in witches' brews because of its power to throw victims into convulsions.

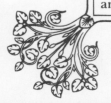

Henna
Lawsonia inermis   sdm
Utilized since earliest times to tint hair, fingernails and skin, orange-brown.

Hollyhock
Alcea rosea   mi
As a gargle, the dried flower tea helps soothe mouth and throat inflammations. Tall majestic flower spikes are covered with double red, pink, purple or yellow blossoms.

Hops
Humulus lupulus   mih
Well known ingredient in beer. Important medicinally for its calming effect. A pillow stuffed with hops flowers is said to overcome insomnia.

Horehound
Marrubium vulgare   m
Horehound candies, once the sovereign remedy for coughs, are still remembered by some. Infusion is useful for weak stomach, lack of appetite and persistent bronchitis.

Hyssop
Hyssopus officinalis   cmih
Decorative plant with a refreshing aromatic scent. Slightly bitter leaves are finely chopped on salad, game meats, soups and stews. Helps digestion. Essential oil used in perfumery.

Hyssop, Hedge
Gratiola officinalis   mp
Formerly used for chronic eczema, scrofula, jaundice and dropsy. Violent purgative: should not be used without medical supervision.

Indian Tobacco. *See* Lobelia.

Jacob's Ladder
Polemonium caeruleum   m
Leaflets are assembled in ladder form. Showy bright blue flowers. Remedy for nervous complaints, headaches and palpitations of the heart.

Jimsonweed. *See* Stramonium.

Joe-Pye Weed
Eupatorium purpureum   m
(Gravelroot). Tall, graceful native of eastern United States. Leaves vanilla-scented when crushed; flowers rosy-purple. Indians and pioneers used it to induce sweating to break fevers. Valuable remedy for kidney problems.

Juniper
Juniperus communis   cmid
Well-known evergreen shrub. Berries stimulate appetite, digestion and other bodily functions.

Lady's Mantle
Alchemilla vulgaris   m
Graceful low-growing herb. Round velvety leaves and delicate sprays of chartreuse flowers are lovely in rock gardens or low borders. Its astringent quality has earned it great esteem through the ages for treating wounds, diarrhea and excessive menstruation.

Lambs Ear, Woolly
Stachys byzantina   m
Delightful soft, downy foliage resembles lamb's ears in feel and appearance. Silvery appearance is ideal for contrasting and grey gardens. Formerly used to bandage wounds.

Lambs Quarters
Chenopodium album   cm
Common weed, popular as a potherb. Young tender plants are a pleasant spinach substitute when boiled and served with butter. Also served raw in salads. Rich source of vitamins A and C.

Lantern Plant
Physalis alkekengi   cm
Edible berries are borne inside fascinating orange chinese lantern-like calyces. Berries are eaten raw, or in preserves and pies. Recommended for fevers and gout.

Lavender. *See* p. 188.

Lettuce, Wild
Lactuca virosa   m
Dried milky juice, called lactucarium or lettuce opium, was once used to induce sleep and to treat nervous disorders.

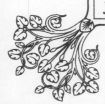

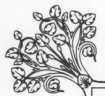

Lily of the Valley
Convallaria majalis   mpd
Pure white, fragrant flowers and pale green foliage. Strengthens and regulates the heart.

Linden
Tilia cordata   tms
(Limeflower). Stately street or lawn trees. Fragrant flowers make a delicious digestive tisane, popular as an after-dinner beverage. Pleasant alternative to aspirin for feverish colds, for it reduces temperature and helps promote sleep. Facial steam of linden tea improves skin circulation and smoothes wrinkles.

Lobelia
Lobelia inflata   mp
(Indian Tobacco). In small doses lobelia acts as a stimulant, especially on the respiratory system. In larger doses it acts as a nerve depressant, and is useful for asthma and whooping cough. Should not be used without medical supervision as excessive doses can cause severe depression.

Lobelia, Great
Lobelia siphilitica   m
Showy native of the United States with large blue flower spikes. Employed by Indians in combination with mayapple (*Podophyllum peltatum*) roots to treat venereal disease.

Loosestrife, Purple
Lythrum salicaria   m
Once highly esteemed for curing chronic diarrhea and dysentery. Rarely used in medicine now, loosestrife is grown for the beauty it lends to the garden.

Lovage
Levisticum officinale   cmit
Leaves possess excellent flavouring qualities for soups, stews and casseroles. Can replace meat and bones in soups because it gives the impression a complete soup extract has been added.

Mallow, Musk
Malva moschata   m
Handsome rose-mauve flowers attract honey bees. Leaves emit faint musky odour, especially during warm weather or when drawn through the hand. Useful for inflammations of the alimentary, urinary and respiratory systems.

Marjoram, Common
Origanum vulgare   mcd
(Wild Oregano). Medicinal variety of oregano lacking true oregano's familiar aroma and flavour. Used for upset stomach, headache, cough, and diarrhea. Also as gargle for mouth and throat inflammations. Handsome purple or pink flowers attract honeybees. See also p. 188.

Marshmallow
Althaea officinalis   m
Noted for its soothing qualities. For irritations and inflammations of the skin, throat, eyes, lungs and urinary organs.

Melilot
Melilotus officinalis   mh
(Sweet Clover). Important forage crop. Medicinally, it prevents blood clotting. Salve or poultice is useful for swellings, boils, arthritis and rheumatism.

Mint. *See* p. 189.

Motherwort
Leonurus cardiaca   m
Especially valuable for female weakness and disorders. Helps calm the entire nervous system. Old remedy for strengthening the heart.

Mugwort
Artemisia vulgaris   m
Bitter flower buds add an interesting touch to rich meat, poultry or fish dishes, and improve the digestibility of these foods. In early England dried leaves and flowertops were commonly steeped for tea.

Mulberry
Morus nigra   cm
Handsome tree bearing sweet, juicy berries that make fine conserves and drinks,

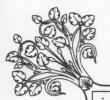

including mulberry wine. Rootbark decoction is a traditional remedy for tapeworms. Hardy in southwestern Ontario and coastal British Columbia, Canada.

Mullein
Verbascum thapsus m
Striking yellow flower stalks rise from a woolly leaf base. Good remedy for coughs, hoarseness and bronchitis.

Myrtle
Myrtus communis hcms
Classic evergreen shrub from the Mediterranean. Fragrant white flowers and leaves are unique in potpourris and sachets. Spicy leaves can be used in cooking like bay leaf. Lovely house plant.

Nettle, Stinging
Urtica dioica cndi
Drying or cooking removes stinging effect of the leaves. Leaves can be used in salt-reduced diets, as they contain a salt which is not a burden on the system. Cooked young shoots, rich in iron, are commonly eaten as tonic spring greens.

New Jersey Tea
Ceanothus americanus mtd
(Red Root). Used as a tea substitute during the American Revolution. Indians made a wash for skin problems including skin cancer and venereal sores. A good gargle for mouth and throat sores.

Oregano, Wild. *See* Marjoram, Common.

Parsley. *See* p. 190.

Pasque Flower
Anemone pulsatilla m
Pretty rock garden plant with masses of purple flowers appearing early in spring. Valuable in correcting membrane disorders of the respiratory and digestive passages.

Passion Fruit
Passiflora edulis cm
Unusual vine bearing spectacular star-like lavender flowers. Edible purple fruits possess pleasant flavour. Used as table fruit and in sherbet, jam, and beverages.

Pennyroyal
Mentha pulegium cmt
Strong minty odour. Used in earlier times to flavour puddings and sauces. Tea is still used today to ease headache. Has insect-repelling properties.

Pepper, Cayenne
Capsicum annuum (Longum) cm
Hot, pungent pods are indispensable in Mexican, Indonesian and Italian dishes. An insect repellent spray for the garden is made with ground pods mixed with water and a little soap.

Periwinkle, Madagascar
Catharanthus roseus m
(Vinca Rosea). Source of several anti-cancer alkaloids used in treating leukemia and other forms of cancer. Has been employed as a tea for diabetics. Flowers rose, salmon, pink or white.

Pimpernel
Anagallis arvensis m
Ancient reputation for treating depression, melancholy, and allied mental disorders. Scarlet, white or blue flowers close when bad weather is imminent, earning the name "weatherglass."

Pitcher Plant
Sarracenia purpurea m
Fascinating insect-eating plant. Colourful pitcher-like leaves with arching hoods and honey scent attract and trap small insects. North American Indians used an infusion of the rootstock for smallpox. Bog plant.

Pleurisy Root
Asclepias tuberosa m
Bright orange-red flowers. Roots act specifically on the lungs, assisting expectoration and subduing inflammation. Valuable for all chest complaints, including pleurisy.

Pokeroot
Phytolacca americana chmpd
Pleasant early sping potherb tasting like asparagus. Young unfolded leaves (older

leaves are poisonous) are boiled for 15 minutes and drained. They are simmered in fresh water for 20 minutes; salt and butter added to taste. Powdered roots were used in a poultice by early settlers to treat cancerous ulcers.

Pomegranate, Dwarf
Punica granatum 'Nana' cdm
Showy orange-red fuchsia-like flowers; miniature fruits. Considered an excellent remedy for tapeworms since the time of the Greeks.

Prickly Pear
Opuntia humifusa cm
Interesting cactus. Bears edible fruits (pears) having pleasant, somewhat acid taste. May be eaten raw or dried, first discarding thick skins and seeds. A nutritious and stimulating sauce, similar to apple sauce, is prepared by boiling in water for 10-12 hours, then allowing to ferment a little.

Privet
Ligustrum vulgare dm
Excellent hedge plant. Clippings yield yellow or gold dyes. Astringent decoction of leaves or bark is helpful for diarrhea, sore throat and certain skin problems.

Queen Anne's Lace
Daucus carota m
(Wild Carrot). Infusion is considered valuable in the treatment of dropsy, chronic kidney disease and bladder afflictions. Leaves applied with honey soothe external sores and ulcers.

Ramsons
Allium ursinum cm
(Wild Garlic). Strong garlic odour and flavour. Whole plant, collected in summer and autumn, is used fresh like garlic in salads. Helpful for arteriosclerosis, lack of appetite and diarrhea.

Rauwolfia
Rauvolfia serpentina mp
Famous tranquillizer plant of India, where for 3,000 years it has been used to treat mental illness. Long ignored by the West until the 1950s. Today highly valued in medicine for its powerful hypnotic and sedative properties.

Red Root. *See* New Jersey Tea.

Restharrow
Ononis spinosa m
Good diuretic lacking usual harmful side-effects. Effective for dropsy, rheumatism, gout, and bladder and kidney disorders.

Rose, Dog
Rosa canina cmt
Fruits (rosehips) are 20 times richer in vitamin C than oranges. Used in preserves, sauces and tea.

Rosemary. *See* p. 191.

Rue
Ruta graveolens mhnd
Pungent bitter leaves used sparingly in stews, salads, sandwiches and vegetable juice. Two leaves chewed will quickly relieve nervous headache. In early times judges relied on fresh sprigs of rue to repel fleas brought into court by prisoners.

Rupturewort
Herniaria glabra m
Valuable for urinary problems as it increases sodium and urea emission without increasing urine flow. Helps to relieve kidney and bladder pains.

Saffron, Meadow. *See* Colchicum.

Sage. *See* p. 192.

St. Johnswort
Hypericum perforatum md
Noted for its calming effect; valuable for nervous disorders such as insomnia, depression and bed-wetting. The oil has remarkable soothing and healing action when rubbed into painful joints and strained muscles. Bright yellow flowers.

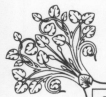

Sarsaparilla
Aralia hispida m
Woody perennial native to New England. Bark and roots have special action on the kidneys. Of merit for dropsy, gravel and other urinary diseases.

Sassafras
Sassafras albidum timd
Tree native to the United States. Spicy root bark is used to make delicious tonic tea. Used in soaps and perfumes and to flavour tobacco, root beer, dentifrices and chewing gum.

Sea-Onion
Ornithogalum caudatum m
A fascinating onion-like medicinal herb. Known as the 'pregnant onion,' for bulges develop on its sides where eventually "baby" bulbs burst through the skin. Leaves or bulblets are made into ointments for treating persistent sores.

Shepherds Purse
Capsella bursa-pastoris m
Considered one of the most important drug plants. Infusion is excellent for stopping internal and external hemorrhages. Recommended for excessive and difficult menstruation.

Skullcap
Scutellaria lateriflora m
Effective, reliable remedy for headache and neuralgia. Good sedative for insomnia, restlessness, hysteria and convulsions.

Soapwort
Saponaria officinalis hm
Excellent shampoos, skin rinses and washes for delicate fabrics are made by steeping roots in water. Lathers like soap when agitated. As a skin rinse it helps relieve itchiness.

Speedwell
Veronica officinalis m
Infusion is useful for coughs and catarrh. As a lotion it is effective for skin eruptions and slow-healing wounds. Low creeping herb with pale blue flowers.

Stramonium
Datura stramonium mp
(Jimson Weed). Sometimes given for spasmodic coughing and bronchial asthma. Leaves steeped in water are said to induce visions along with giddiness and delirium. Fatal in large doses.

Strawberry, Wild
Fragaria vesca cm
Infusion of leaves and rootstock is effective for diarrhea, dysentery and problems of the urinary tract. Especially useful for convalescents and children. Cultivated varieties are much less potent medicinally.

Sunflower
Helianthus annuus chim
Familiar large yellow sunflowers are a favourite of children. Valued for its highly nutritious seeds eaten roasted or raw.

Tansy
Tanacetum vulgare cmdh
Pretty yellow button flowers were once used by North American Indians to induce abortion. Now used in various cosmetic preparations. Repels ants from counters or around baseboards.

Teasel, Fullers
Dipsacus sativus cmi
Comb-like flowerheads were once an important article of commerce for raising nap on woollen cloth. Excellent in dried arrangements. Leaf basins collect water which is valued as an eyewash.

Thistle, Blessed
Cnicus benidictus mt
Main medicinal value is as a tonic, particularly for the digestive system. Said to improve blood purification and circulation, thereby helping to strengthen the brain and memory.

Thistle, Milk
Silybum marianum mc
Striking plant. Its glossy leaves are painted with veins of creamy white which, according to tradition, originated from the milk of

the Virgin which once fell upon a plant. Medicinal use similar to blessed thistle.

Thyme. *See* p. 193.

Toadflax
Linaria vulgaris   m
Pretty yellow and orange flowers are like miniature snapdragons. Juice or tea is recommended for sore eyes, skin irritations, and hemorrhoids.

Tobacco
Nicotiana tabacum   hnm
Tobacco of commerce. Has been used to relax spasms, relieve local pain and constipation. A good insect-repelling spray is made by steeping leaves in water for 24 hours, then adding a little soap as a wettening agent.

Tobacco, Wild
Nicotiana rustica   nhm
Originally grown and smoked by North American Indians. Now the chief source of nicotine sulphate, an important insecticide for the control of aphids, thrips, whiteflies and mites.

Valerian
Valeriana officinalis   mi
Excellent sedative action. Widely used to allay pain, nervous unrest, migraine, neuralgia and insomnia.

Vervain
Verbena officinalis   mt
An aphrodisiac, said to 'secure the favour of the ladies.' Historically associated with sorcerers and witches. Slightly bitter tisane is of very old usage as a digestive and sedative nightcap.

Vinca Rosea. *See* Periwinkle.

Violet, Sweet
Viola odorata   mhis
Old garden favourite. Sweet-scented, deep violet flowers are delightful candied as decoration for cakes, puddings and ice cream. Violet tea or syrup is a good cough medicine. Important source of perfume.

Witch-Hazel
Hamamelis virginiana   m
Astringent leaf and bark preparations are very effective in checking internal and external hemorrhages. Ointment is a good general remedy for cuts, burns and inflammations.

Woad
Isatis tinctoria   dm
Woad was the main source of blue dye in Europe, until the introduction of indigo in the 17th century.

Woodruff, Sweet
Galium odoratum   hmi
Sweet scented dried leaves, their scent resembling vanilla, are delightful in potpourris and sachets. An exhilarating German punch called 'Maibowle,' made by steeping leaves in white wine, is traditionally drunk on the first of May. Neat compact plants, covered with white flowers in spring.

Wormseed. *See* Epazote.

Wormwood
Artemisia absinthium   cmit
Intensely bitter leaves were an important ingredient in absinthe, vermouth, and other liqueurs. Has great reputation for stimulating the appetite and improving digestion. One of the oldest known remedies for worms.

Yarrow
A. millefolium   mst
Yarrows are impressive all-round natural remedies. Owing to their bitter principles, they have the reputation as general fortifiers, helping to build the body's natural resistance. They improve digestion, circulation, and the functions of the liver, gall bladder, and kidneys. They are valuable wound herbs for cuts and make excellent cosmetic lotions for cleansing and beautifying the skin.

Yerba Mate
Ilex paraguariensis tm
Maté tea is a popular South American beverage. More stimulating than coffee or tea but contains little caffeine. Very rich in vitamins and minerals. Has valuable restorative and sustaining properties.

Yucca
Yucca glauca ihm
Roots contain two per cent saponin, a soapy substance valuable in shampoos, leaving a fine sheen to hair. Excellent for washing delicate fabrics. Easy to use; chopped roots are soaked in water and stirred to a lather. Spectacular towering spikes of creamy white flowers.

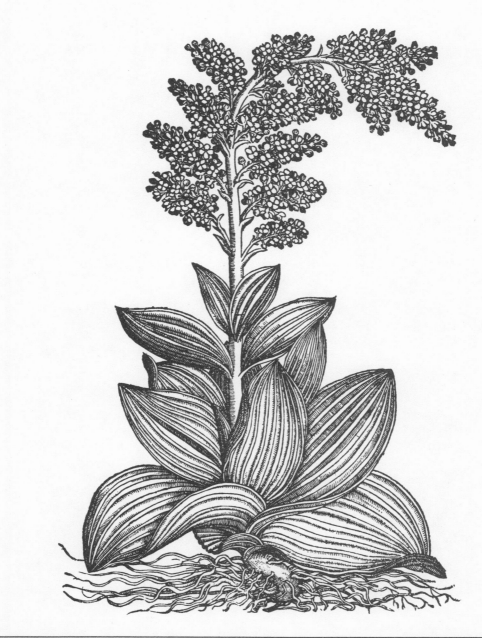

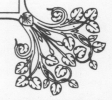

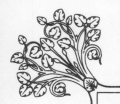

Bibliography & Notes on Sources

The Accomplished Housewife—Receipts in Physick, London, 1754

Albertus Magnus or Egyptian Secrets, 1880, New York.

Avery's Almanack, 1857, Saint John, New Brunswick.

Bill Wannan's Folk Medicine, 1970, Melbourne, Australia (Hill of Content Publishing Co. Pty.)

The Book of Household Management, Mrs Isabella Beeton, 1861, London.

A Book of Simples, 1908, London (Chiswicke Press). Original Still-room book 1750.

Brews and Potions, compiled by Maurice Richards, 1968, London (Hugh Evelyn Ltd).

Brockville Almanac, 1866, 1867, Brockville Ontario.

Buckeye Cookery, 1881, Minneapolis, Minnesota.

The Canada Farmer, Toronto, Jan.-Dec. 1847, also 1864-76.

The Canadian Farmer's Almanac and Memorandum Book, 1850, Sherbrooke, C.E.

The Canadian Home Cook Book, 1877, published by the Ladies of Toronto. Hunter Rose. Ontario Reprint Society 1970. Coles Publishing 1971.

A Collection of Receipts in Cookery, Physick and Surgery, Mrs Mary Kettilby, 1749, London

The Compleat Housewoman, Hannah Wooley, 1711

The Compleat Vermin Killer and Useful Pocket Companion, 1778, Dublin.

The Complete Family Piece and Country Gentleman and Farmer's Best Guide, 1741, London.

Curious Old Cookery Receipts Including Simples for Simple Ailments, 1891, London.

Delights for Ladies, Sir Hugh Platt, 1609, London.

The Domestic Physician and Traveller's Medical Companion, compiled ...by a Physician, 1845, Toronto (Payne).

Dr Case's New Recipe Book, 1882, New York

Dr Chases's Recipes or Information for Everyone, 1867, 1880, 1892, Ann Arbor, Michigan.

The English Physician, Nicholas Culpeper, to which is added **The Family Physician** by Dr Parkins, 1814, London. Original title: English Physitian or An Astro Physical Discourse of the Vulgar Herbs of this Nation, London, 1652.

Egyptian Secrets. See **Albertus Magnus.**

The Family Magazine, 1741, London.

The Family Manual Containing Things Worth Knowing, 1845, New York.

The Family Nurse or Companion of the Frugal Housewife, Lydia Maria Child, Boston, 1837.

The Family Oracle of Health, Economy, Medicine and Good Living, 1825, London.

The Family Physician and the Farmer's Companion, Syracuse, New York, 1840.

The Family Physician. See **The English Physician.**

The Family Receipt Book—Contains Thirty Valuable and Simple Receipts for the Cure of Most the Usual Complaints, 1825, New York.

The Farmer's Advocate, 1875-1924, London, Ontario.

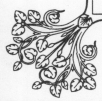
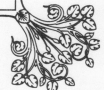

Farmer's Directory and Housekeeper's Assistant, 1851, Toronto.

Farmers and Housekeepers Cyclopaedia, 1977, Trumansburg, N.Y. (The Crossing Press).

Foxfire I, edited by Brooks Elliot Wigginton, 1972 (Doubleday).

The Frugal Housewife, Lydia Maria Child, 1831, Boston.

The Hearthstone, 1883, Laura Carter Holloway, Philadelphia.

An Historical Almanac of Canada, Lena Newman, 1967, Toronto, (McClelland and Stewart).

The Home Cook Book, Toronto, 1884.

The Household Book of Practical Receipts, London, 1871.

The Housekeeper's Almanac, 1842, New York

The Housekeeper's Guide, 1868, Cincinnati, Ohio.

The Housekeeper's Pocket Book—Everyone Their Own Physician, Circa 1750.

The Improved Housewife, 1864, Hartford.

Inglenook Doctor Book, 1911, first reprinting 1975, Illinois (Brethern Publishing House).

John Stoner's Sympathy—A Collection of Excellent Remedies and Recipes for the Cure of Various Diseases of Persons and Cattle, Ohio, 1867.

Kentucky Superstitions, Daniel and Lucy Thomas, 1920, Princeton, N.J. (Princeton University Press).

Ladies Indispensable Assistant—Being a Companion for the Sister, Mother and Wife—A Great Variety of Valuable Recipes forming a complete system of Family Medicine, Thus enabling Each Person to become His or Her Own Physician, 1851, N.Y.

The Lady's Annual Register and Housewife's Memorandum Book, 1838, Boston.

A Little Book of Conceited Secrets and Delights for Ladies, Moira Meighn, 1928, London and Boston (The Medici Society).

The Long Lost Friend, John George Hohman, 1856

Lotions and Potions, the National Federal of Women's Institutes, England.

McMillan's New Brunswick Almanac and Register, 1866, Saint John, New Brunswick (McAlpine Directory Co.)

Merchant and Farmer's Almanack, 1855, Saint John, New Brunswick.

Moore's Almanack, Francis Moore, London, 1912.

Murray's Elements of Cookery, circa 1850, London.

The New Cook Book, 1906, Grace E. Denison, Toronto.

New England Rarities Discovered, John Josselyn, 1672, London.

New Family Receipt Book, 1815, London.

A Number of Receipts for Curing Different Diseases in Man and Beast, 1855.

The People's Almanac, Montreal, 1855.

The People's Home Library, Book 1, **The People's Home Medical Book,** T.J. Ritter, 1916, Cleveland (R.C. Barum & Co.).

The People's Manual, 1848, Worcester, Mass.

A Plain Plantain—Country Wines, Dishes and Herbal Cures from a 17th C. Household Receipt Book, arranged by Russell George Alexander, Sussex (St. Dominic's Press).

Primitive Physick: Or An Easy and Natural Method of Curing Most Diseases, Reverend John Wesley, 1747 (T. Tyre).

A Queen's Delight—A Right Knowledge of making Perfumes and Distilling the Most Excellent Waters, 1671, London.

The Receipt Book of Mrs Ann Blencowe, 1694, London. Limited edition published 1925 (The Adelphi Guy Chapman).

Six Hundred Receipts Worth their Weight in Gold, 1890, Philadelphia.

Stere Itt Well—A book of Medieval Refinements, Recipes and Remedies from a Manuscript in Samuel Pepys's Library, 1972, Cambridge (Cornmarket Reprints).

Texas Folk Medicine, 1970, John Q. Anderson, Austin, Texas (Encini Press).

The United States Practical Receipt Book, 1844, Philadelphia.

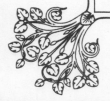

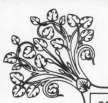

Universal Receipt Book Containing Scarce, Curious and Valuable Receipts and Choice Secrets by a Society of Gentlemen in New York, 1814.

REFERENCE BOOKS

American Indian Medicine, Vergil Vogel, 1970 (University of Oklahoma Press).

Blacks Medical Dictionary, 1976, New York, (Harper and Row Publishers, Inc.).

Choosing, Planting and Cultivating Herbs, Philippa Back, 1977, (Keats Publishing Inc.).

Cures and Remedies—The Country Way, Robin Page, 1978, London, (David and Poynter Ltd.).

Encyclopedia of Superstitions, 1961, London, (Hutchinson and Co.).

Familiar Medical Quotations, edited by Maurice B. Strauss, 1968, (Little Brown and Co.).

Familiar Quotations, John Bartlett, 1968 edition, Boston (Little, Brown and Co.).

Folklore of the Teeth, Leo Kanner, 1928, New York (The MacMillan Co.).

The Forgotten Art of Growing, Gardening and Cooking with Herbs, Richard Bacon, 1972, Yankee Books

Funk and Wagnall's Standard Dictionary of Folklore, Mythology and Legend, 1972, London, (New English Library).

Grandmother's Secrets, Jean Palaiseul, 1976, (Penguin Books).

A Guide to the Medicinal Plants of the United States, Arnold and Connie Krochmal, 1978 (Quadrangle, The New York Times Book Co.).

Herb Gardens of Delight, Adelma Simmons, 1974 (Hawthorne Books Inc.).

The Home Book of Proverbs, Maxims and Familiar Phrases, selected and arranged by Burton Stevenson, 1948, New York (The MacMillan Company).

The Home Book of Quotations, selected and arranged by Burton Stevenson, 1953, New York (Dodd, Mead and Company).

Magic of Herbs, Mrs. C.F. Leyel, 1926 (London, Butler and Tanner Ltd.).

Medicines from the Earth—A Guide to Healing Plants, edited by William A.R. Thomson, 1978, Maidenhead, England (McGraw-Hill Book Co.).

A Modern Herbal (two volumes), Mrs M. Grieve, 1971 (Dover Publications.).

The Oxford Dictionary of Quotations, Geoffrey Cambridge, 1953, London (Oxford University Press).

Notes on Sources

The remedies and advice identified in this book as Texas remedies are from *Texas Folk Medicine*; Appalachian Remedies are from *Foxfire*. *Bill Wannan's Folk Medicine* was the source for information from the *Australian Household Manual*, *The Emigrant's Guide to Australia*, the *Kandy Koola Cook Book* and the *Kookaburra Cookery Book*. *A Little Book of Conceited Secrets and Delights for Ladies* contained material originally published in *The Good Housewife's Jewell*, *The True Preserver*, *The Garden of Pleasant Flowers* and *The Art of Cookery Made Plain and Easy by a Lady*. Excerpts from *Polygraphices* can be found in *Lotions and Potions* and for early Anglo-Saxon remedies see *Brews and Potions*.

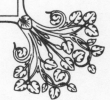

Herb Suppliers

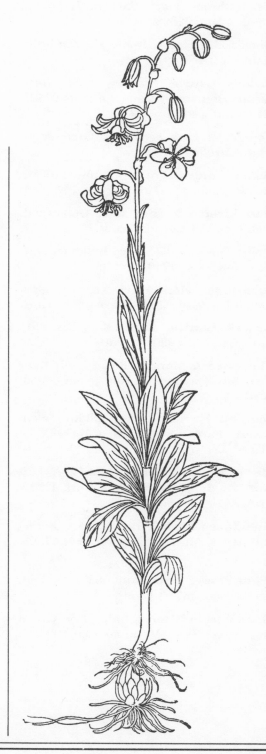

Ashby's Garden Centre & Nursery, R.R. 2, Highway 35, Cameron, Ontario, Canada. Plants

Carobil Farm, Church Rd., R.D. 1, Brunswick, Maine 04011. Scented and other geraniums.

Carroll Gardens, Box 310, Westminster, Maryland 21157. Plants.

Comstock, Ferre & Co., 263 Main St., Wethersfield, Connecticut 06109. Seeds.

Culpeper Ltd., 21 Bruton St., London W1X 7DA; or 59 Ebury St., London SW1 ONZ; or 14 Crystal Palace Parade SE 19.

Gurney Seed Co., Yankton, South Dakota 57078.

Joseph Harris Co., Moreton Farm, Rochester, New York 14624. Seeds.

Hemlock Hill Herb Farm, Hemlock Hill Rd., Litchfield, Connecticut 06759. Plants.

The Herb Cottage, Washington National Cathedral, Washington, D.C. 20016. Seeds.

The Herbary and Potpourri Shop, Box 543, Childs Homestead Rd., Orleans, Massachusetts 02653. Plants and seeds.

Madge Hooper, FRHS., Stoke-Lacy Herb Farm, Bromyard, Herefordshire.

Howe Hill Herbs, Camden, Maine 04843. Plants.

J. H. Hudson, Seedsman, Box 1058, Redwood City, California 94064.

Logee's Greenhouses, 55 North St., Danielson, Connecticut 06239. Plants.

McFarland House Garden Shop and Greenhouses, 5923 Exchange St., McFarland, Wisconsin 53558. Plants.

Meadowbrook Herb Garden, Wyoming, Rhode Island 02898.

Monk's Hill Herbs, Route 17, Winthrop, Maine 04364.

Nichols Garden Nursery, 1190 North Pacific Highway, Albany, Oregon 97321. Plants and seeds.

George W. Park Seed Co., Greenwood, South Carolina 29646.

Pellett Gardens, Atlantic, Iowa 50022. Honey plants.

Otto Richter & Sons Ltd., Goodwood, Ont. L0C 1A0, Canada. Seeds.

Stokes Seeds, 1017 Stokes Building, Buffalo, New York 14240.

Sunnybrook Herb Farm Nursery, Mayfield Rd., Chesterland, Ohio 44026. Plants.

Taylor's Garden, 1535 Lone Oak Rd., Vista, California 92083. Plants.

Thompson & Morgan, Box 24, 401 Kennedy Blvd., Somerdale, New Jersey 08083. Seeds.

Tool Shed Nursery, Turkey Hill Rd., Salem Centre, Purdy's Station, New York 12865. Plants.

Martin Viette Nurseries, Route 25A, East Norwich, Long Island, New York 11732. Plants.

Well-Sweep Herb Farm, 317 Mt. Bethel Rd., Port Murray, New Jersey 07865. Plants.

White Flower Farm, Route 63, Litchfield, Connecticut 06759. Plants.

Wide World of Herbs, Ltd., 11 St. Catherine Street East, Montreal, Canada. Seeds.

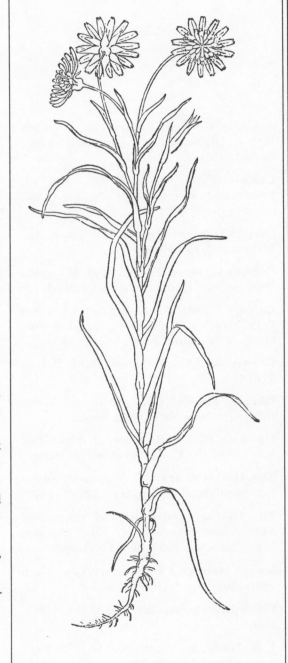

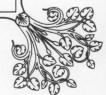

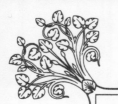

Apothecaries' Weights and Equivalents

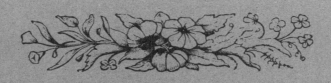

Apothecaries' Weight	Abbrev.	Equivalents	Metric Equivalent
1 Grain	gr.	0.002 286 oz. av.*	64.799 mg
1 Scruple	sc. ap.	20 gr.	1.296 0 g
1 Drachm	dr. ap.	3 sc.	3.887 9 g
1 Ounce	oz. ap.	8 dr. ap. 1 oz. t.** 1.097 oz. av.	31.103 g
1 Pound	lb. ap.	12 oz. ap. 0.822 9 lb. av.	373.24 g

* avoirdupois system
** troy system

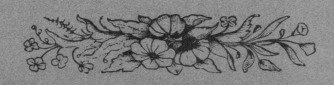

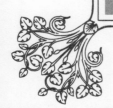

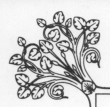

Personal Receipts

_____

_____

_____

_____

_____

_____

_____

_____

_____

_____

_____

_____

_____

_____

_____

_____

_____

_____

_____

_____

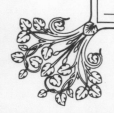
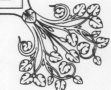

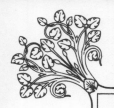

Personal Receipts

_____

_____

_____

_____

_____

_____

_____

_____

_____

_____

_____

_____

_____

_____

_____

_____

_____

_____

_____

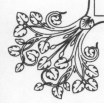
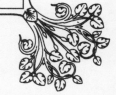

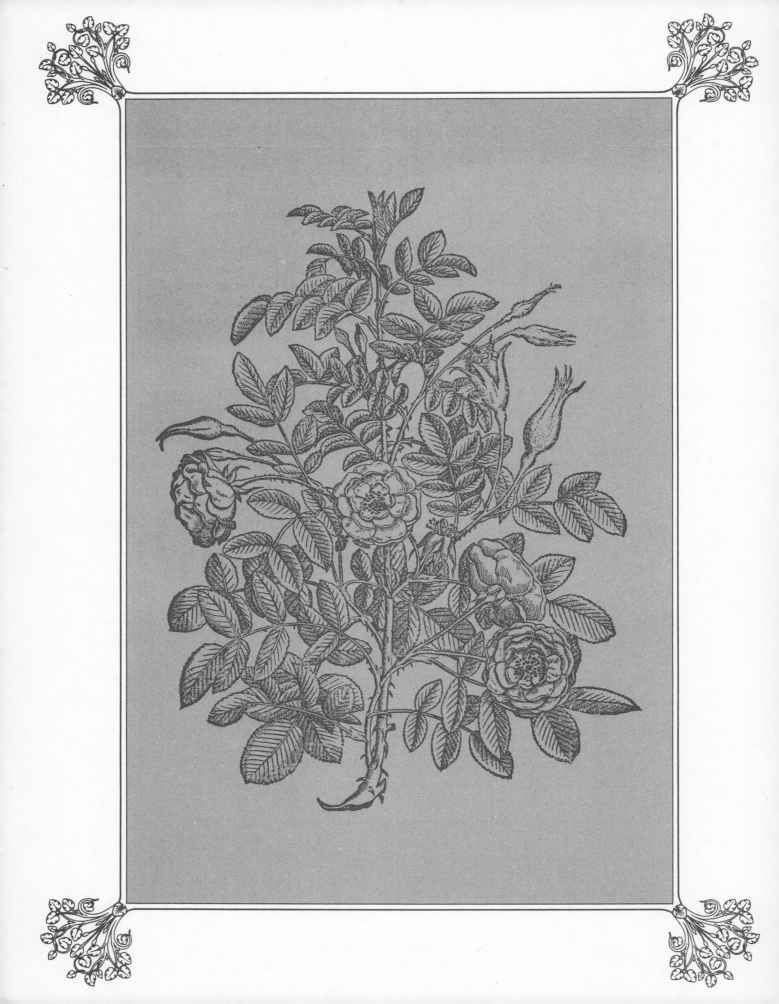